Pregnancy

F🛇R MEN

The whole 9 months

Mark Woods

This edition first published in Great Britain 2010 by
Crimson Publishing, a division of Crimson Business Ltd
Westminster House
Kew Road
Richmond
Surrey
TW9 2ND

A catalogue record for this book is available from the British Library.

ISBN 978 1 90541 0620

Printed and bound in the UK by Asford Colour Press Ltd, Gosport, Hants

Acknowledgements

I owe a huge debt of gratitude to all the Dads who contributed to this book. Your honesty, and in many cases bravery, will not go unrecorded in the annals of male history. I salute you.

Many thanks also to the fantastic team at Crimson Publishing including Beth Bishop, Holly Ivins, Sally Rawlings, Lucy Smith and especially David Lester. Thanks also go to Simon Fitzmaurice for the cartoons and Carol Farley for spreading the word.

Thanks to Rebecca Winfield for the sage advice, Caroline Millar for her invaluable research, Sara Warren for casting an experienced midwife's eye over the detail, and my Mum and Dad for deciding that six kids just wasn't enough.

But mainly thank you to my amazing little boy Stan for being so beautiful and to my wife Sarah for being even more beautiful and only letting the fact that I spent six months shut in a small room get on her nerves very occasionally.

To Sarah, Stan and the wee one on the way, with love.

December 2013

Dearest little brother,

I bought this book when Tash was expecting Noah. As a first time father I found it really helpful. This isn't a new copy, it's the actual copy I read and I really wanted you to have it and READ it!! You read it month-to-month so you can get an understanding of both what little "Krisaniel" is doing and also what Krista is going through. Sorry I never got it to you sooner but I really do think you will enjoy it.

As a new father to a father-to-be let me tell you are in for an amazing year in 2014. Enjoy every minute of it because your life will never be the same. You are going to be an AWESOME Dad!

Love you Big Bro xxx

About the author

Mark Woods has covered national and international stories for the UK's premier news agency, the Press Association; helped to bring a multi-million pound TV company to its knees and is now a writer and ideas man for the charity Comic Relief.

He lives in south west London with his wife and son Stanley.

Contents

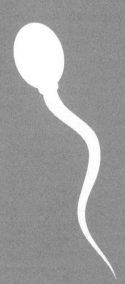

INTRODUCTION

A generation or two ago you were more likely to see a fully grown llama at a birth than the father of the child. Now more than 90% of deliveries have the dad-to-be in attendance. That's a profound change, not least for llamas who have been all but banished from the scene. With this shift has also come a gradual increase in the involvement of the father in the pregnancy itself.

In the main, this change has been welcomed and driven by modern man; as the nature of relationships have changed for the better, so has the desire of many men to be involved in arguably the most important event that a couple can share together.

Preparing for such a momentous period isn't easy. All pregnancies and indeed births, are different, but despite this, over the years some excellent books have been put together to give women the blow-by-blow information they need on carrying and delivering a baby. While these books are perfectly pitched at the mother, they often fail to take in a vital facet of the male psyche, namely the fact that we don't really properly listen to anything, unless it's about us. It's an unattractive trait I'll admit, but then again it's got quite a few to keep it company, hasn't it?

Of course the central characters of any book on pregnancy are the main protagonists in the drama, the mother and the child. But with the increasing role of the father in the whole nine months, it's only right that they get a guide book that is written by them and for them.

This is what *Pregnancy for Men* aims to do. How? By delivering factual information in a straightforward, logical way and crucially, *crucially*, taking every single opportunity that presents itself to execute a puerile or tastefully questionable comment in order to produce the lubricant that will allow this or any kind of material to slide into a man's brain – humour.

Please don't misunderstand me, it's my sincere hope that this is a very comprehensive and useful book that will provide men with just about everything they need to know about making a baby from conception to cord cutting (and all of the information has been checked by an experienced midwife). But it's got quite a few gags in it too, that's all I'm saying.

There is a distinct possibility that this is being purchased by a woman for a man, most likely her partner. As we all know, men don't generally buy self-help books for the simple reason that we don't need any help whatsoever, unless we are trying to find something in a drawer or cupboard of course. If you happen to be a woman, rest assured that within these pages you are held in the highest regard, revered almost, for what you go through to produce a baby. You may even find the way the information is communicated here a refreshing alternative to the many, often daunting, pregnancy guides you have no doubt got stacked beside your bed at this very moment.

You are most welcome.

I structured this book in month-by-month chapters because throughout the birth of my own son I became so confused by the week-to-week method often employed that I began to ensure I was always wearing presentable socks – so positive was I that they would be on show at some point as I once again called on the use of my toes to help me work things out.

As in life, things don't fall neatly into designated timeframes throughout pregnancy, but I've done my very best to ensure that most of what is contained within each month is roughly relevant to that part of the journey.

To avoid confusion I refer to the baby as 'he' throughout this book, for no other reason than it is one letter shorter than she and as you are soon to discover, once you have a baby saving even one 's' worth of time is worth doing.

I hope you enjoy reading *Pregnancy for Men* and find it useful too – I certainly did and can only apologise to my poor wife that I only knew about 5% of what it covers when she was pregnant. I promise that when we have our next one I'll help you out much more.

I loved researching for this book, interviewing other Dads for it and writing it.

Most of all though I love being a Dad and I'm certain you will too.

Good luck in getting there.

PROLOGUE
Making a baby

Before the bumps and the birth plan; before the midwives and the morning sickness; even before the chronic constipation and the crazy cravings – there's making the baby. What could you possibly need to know that could make this gloriously perfect little spell in your life any better?

Well, as ever, the 21st century has managed to complicate the uncomplicatable; to add a soupçon of angst to what was once the most beautifully simple of recipes.

If you've negotiated it already, very, very many congratulations, you are on your way to the best, most overwhelming experience of your life. If you're still trying your little heart out to make it happen, here's a very quick jaunt through the ins and outs of making a baby today.

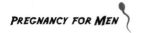

Years hoping not – days hoping so

It's entirely fitting that in a world where immediate gratification is king, we expect to conceive a child the very instant we cease doing everything within our power to stop that very occurrence from taking place.

With more than 3.5 million women in the UK taking the pill at any one time, it is the single most used form of contraception by some distance. This explains why a study by of all places the BBC's *Country File* [1] – yes that's right, John Craven talking about sex – found that so high are the levels of oestrogen flushing into the nation's rivers via sewage works, that half male fish in lowland England are developing female characteristics. Many of the affected fish were rendered sterile or had even begun to develop eggs in their testes. At least one poor specimen was caught pulling the entire box set of *Sex and the City* behind him on a piece of weed.

Tragic.

What's even more alarming, unless you're a boy carp with boobs of course, is that the pill has also been found to change women's taste in men. Researchers have discovered that women who are taking the pill prefer looking at images of the more macho types among us, with strong jaw lines and prominent cheekbones. Women not taking the pill tended to fancy men with more feminine, softer physical features.

The above findings indicate that as women who take the pill cannot become pregnant, they are subconsciously attracted to sexy, macho geezers, rather than to men who are more likely to make a sensible long-term mate. Which is another way of saying that if your partner chose you for your rugged good looks while she was on the pill, there's a chance she might start to regret it the day after she stops taking it.

Having firmly established that oral contraception of the female kind is a potent and powerful beast, it's little wonder that the consensus among medical professionals is that your partner should stop taking it a good month or two before you seriously try to conceive. That little cushion comes in handy for many men. We can wait a little while, oh yes, just to get our eye in as it were, but then we really do expect things to click into place pretty damn sharpish.

Of course this need for breeding speed isn't just down to rank impatience, or indeed the fragility of the male ego; there's another, more tangible and undeniable pressure that means for many of us, time is of the essence from the moment we make the joint decision to start a family: in the UK we are having our first baby later and later. Statistics show that there are now more first-time mothers in the 30–34 age group than there are in the 25–29 bracket. When you consider that according to the Human Fertilisation and Embryology Authority, at 35 women are half as fertile as when they are 25, and at 40 they are half as fertile again as when they were 35 – it's little wonder that it's taking us longer to conceive.

The pain and suffering of genuine infertility, however, is thankfully still fairly rare – the National Health Service (NHS) estimates that of 100 couples trying to conceive naturally:

> 20 will conceive within one month

> 70 will conceive within six months

> 85 will conceive within one year

> 90 will conceive within 18 months

> 95 will conceive within two years

(If, by the way, you've added up the numbers on the left and are trying to fathom out why they come to 360 rather than 100, you should perhaps be asking yourself whether children are really a wise move.)

Of course the forces behind the choice to have kids later in life is well chronicled. From financial pressure for the woman to keep working longer, or her personal desire to build a career, to the pair of you just

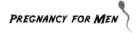

not being ready to face parenthood and give up the high life – more and more of us are waiting longer to swap the nights out for the nappy rash cream.

A final and little-known piece of advice if you are reading this and desperately trying to conceive.

Do you and your partner use personal lubricant? Please excuse the intrusive questioning but recent research has shown that many of the more popular brands seriously inhibit the ability of sperm to get where it needs to go. There are some special sexual lubricants on the market which claim to have overcome this problem, as it were, so it's definitely worth a bit of research before you lube up.

Words from your fellow man:

Colin, 33, father of one: *We made a conscious decision to try when we returned from our honeymoon. Took roughly nine months to get the big 'YES' from the pregnancy test. Didn't happen as quickly as we would have liked to be honest... but we got there in the end!*

David, 34, father of one: *We were 33 and 38, respectively, when we had our first and that sat just fine with me. I'd known I'd wanted children all my adult life, but had also been petrified of having bagsful of regrets when the time actually came. So I made sure in the last couple of years before Lewis arrived that we did our level best to smack the arse out of life. We went on too many holidays, drank too much wine and did too much silly stuff for a couple of our age.*

It took us an increasingly nervous five or six months until we conceived, but it was amazing when it finally happened and life-changing once our son arrived.

Chris, 34, father of one: *My wife, being of a scientific mind (she's a vet), went the clinical route right from the off. Once upon a time you knew a woman was ovulating because after four weeks of disinterest, she was suddenly dragging you to bed. Now a plastic stick tells you when the eggs are on the move. My wife would wee on said stick, it would turn some colour or other and bingo, time to copulate.*

That was one month in. As in, first go. Damn it.

The weird world of gender selection

The sex of your child has always been one of life's great lotteries. Even in this day and age when we manage to find a way to mess about with most things, the numbers still come out pretty equal. In 2004, for instance, 368,000 little boys were born in the UK compared with 348,000 girls.

There are of course a myriad of myths about how you can determine the sex of your baby. First there's only having sex on odd days of the month during a quarter moon for a boy and half moon for a girl. Given that you would need Patrick Moore in the room to work the bloody thing out, it's a method that's probably best avoided – the incessant xylophone playing would put you right off.

Then there's what a woman eats before conception. The story goes that if you want a girl, she should eat lots of magnesium-rich foods such as nuts, soy beans, and leafy green vegetables. If it's a boy you're after, a high-salt diet with plenty of red meat and fizzy beverages is best. So basically it's a healthy diet for a girl and a load of old shite for a boy. Is there any wonder that many of us have to fight off man-boobs from 35 onwards with that kind of start in life?

Surprisingly, there is one theory, one set of instructions, which at least seems to have a semblance of credibility. To understand it you need to know how a baby is made. Pay attention at the back.

Conception occurs when a sperm fertilises an egg. Eggs always carry an X chromosome while sperm can carry an X or a Y chromosome. If an X-carrying sperm fertilises an egg, a baby girl will be conceived and if a Y-carrying sperm fertilises the egg, a baby boy will be conceived. So the gender of the baby is all the man's doing. (Not that long ago many believed that one testicle made boy sperm and the other made girl sperm. Despite the pleasingly symmetrical nature of the theory, it did in time turn out to be... bollocks.)

According to this gender selection theory, boy (Y) sperm travel faster but die more quickly than female (X) sperm. In addition, an acidic environment within the vaginal region is specifically harmful for boy sperm, making conception of a girl more likely.

With these two factors in mind, in order to have a boy, insemination should take place as close as possible to the moment of ovulation so that the thoroughbred-like fast but sickly boy sperm can arrive first and steam ahead straight into the waiting egg. If it's a girl you're after, you should have sex two to three days *before* ovulation – the theory being that although the fast boy sperm get there first, they find nobody at home in the egg department and promptly die. Poor, poor boy sperm.

But don't worry, plodding along behind them like a microscopic cart horse are the girl sperm – and when they get there they have the stamina to hang around for a while in the fallopian tubes until the egg makes its arrival. So, if it's a boy you're after then having sex *as near to* ovulation as possible is key.

But it's not just the timing of the way you have sex that has an effect – it's the position you use too. Shallow penetration, with the sperm deposited close to the entrance of the vagina, favours female conception because the area is more acidic, which kills the weaker boy sperm.

To give the boy sperm a fighting chance to bypass the pool of deadly acid at the entrance, deeper penetration is needed to deposit the sperm at the least acidic area, near the uterus opening. (Interestingly, another conception myth – having sex doggy style to conceive a boy – might not be such rubbish if this theory is to be believed.)

The theory also states that female orgasm favours male sperm because it not only reduces the acid knocking about in the vicinity, but it also makes the entire female reproductive system contract, giving the old slow coach boy sperm the kick up the arse they need to make it all the way.

Of course this theory is far from universally accepted and as with all theories there's a chance it's garbage, but at least you'll have a good time trying to find out. And if you're already pregnant, you can spend time casting your mind back to your performance on that fateful moment to try to guess what it'll be.

What's absolutely certain though is that given the misery that couples unable to conceive endure, the sex of the baby really doesn't matter a jot. What's important is that if you're successful and manage to make a new little life, not only are you a lucky, lucky man, you've also just set a chain of events in motion that will transform you, your partner and the world in which you live forever. Read on Daddy o...

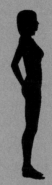

MONTH 1
Is there anybody there?

You've done it. You have played a not so insubstantial part in the creation of a new life. The chances of you doing something more profound, more impactful, more 'God-like' during the entirety of the rest of your life are zero.

Making a baby is an extraordinary thing to do.

Yet everyone's at it, aren't they? Every tired face you see on the way to work in the morning, every foul-mouthed meat head at the football, every chippy teenager on the back seat of the bus – they were all conceived, carried and delivered in one way or another. In fact, every single second that ticks by sees four women give birth to a baby somewhere on the planet. It's no big deal.

And that's the pregnancy paradox you are about to enter into; this most natural of happenings, this most common of occurrences, will rock your world in spectacular fashion.

Of course people close to you will take a lot of interest (mainly women who have been through it or want to be going through it), but all in all the nine months of your first pregnancy are a time when you and your partner are in the most beautiful of bubbles.

It's not all back rubs and belly laughs for sure, the whole experience is laced with an unspeakable fear, the dread that something could go wrong. But as you stand at Month 1, make a little promise to yourself that you'll do your very best to savour every day – because it'll be gone before you know it.

In the beginning was the worm...

We're a funny bunch aren't we? Men I mean.

If I was to ask you to tell me how conception works – not the intercourse bit, everyone is across that one in a big way – but actually what happens from the moment of ejaculation to the precise point when you have a new life on your hands, would you be able to tell me?

The scores of Dads whom I've spoken to in the course of writing this book were to a man-jack, pretty hopeless on that one. Most started off confidently talking about the cervix, took a wrong turn at the uterus and ended up saying the word fallopian a lot, but not much else.

Now, it's entirely possible that I have a particularly uninformed set of friends and acquaintances, and if you knew me, you'd say that was a stone-cold certainty. But I suspect that most people don't really have a bloody clue what happens when a baby is actually conceived by the time they are actually trying to conceive one.

I blame sex education, in particular diagrams such as the one below that the majority of us were shown at some stage of our school careers. It always used to, and indeed still does, look like a skeletal ram eating a carrot to me rather than the cradle of human life.

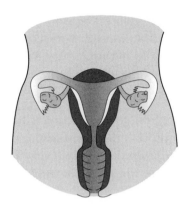

A hungry ram yesterday.

Knowing how the little blighter got there in the first place helps enormously in terms of understanding what's to come in the following nine months of a pregnancy. But before we move on to the main event, let's take a little look at the two central protagonists – the egg and the sperm.

How it actually happens

The ovaries – which are two small organs on either side of the womb (aka the uterus) – are the egg warehouses of the female body. Each and every baby girl is born with up to 450,000 eggs in her ovaries, many of which begin dying off as soon as she enters the world. And there is a steady decrease in number as time goes on. During a woman's fertile years she'll probably release about 400 eggs, beginning with her first period and ending with the menopause.

So far, so double Biology.

Every month, usually during the middle of the menstrual cycle, between one and three eggs start to reach maturity in one of the ovaries. The ripest, juiciest, most prime egg out of the three is then released and in a flash is sucked up by the opening of the nearest fallopian tube – the channel that leads from each ovary to the womb.

This, my friend, is ovulation.

Your average egg survives and can be fertilised for about 12–24 hours after it's released. If it's lucky enough to meet up with a sperm in that time the two can hook up and make a baby. Ahhhh. If not, it ends its journey at the womb, where it disintegrates and is expelled during a period. Ugggh.

Meanwhile, in a ball bag near you, sperm is being produced at a fantastical rate – millions of the microscopic miracles flow off a 24/7 production line, and with 300 million sperm liberated with each ejaculation you can see why your little testicles need to put in the overtime big style.

Working conditions for the heroic duo have to be pretty much spot on and the testicles hang outside your body because they're quite sensitive to temperature. To produce healthy sperm they have to stay at around 34°C and 94°F; that's about 4°C cooler than normal body temperature.

Once sperm is created, it's stored in a coiled tube in the testicle called the epididymis, which if unfurled would measure 40ft long. When the erection alarm bells start ringing as an ejaculation is approaching, the sperm are scooped up and mixed with semen, which helps them travel. They are now ready to have their one and only crack at achieving the goal they were made for – fertilising an egg.

So, having acquainted ourselves with the stars of the show, let's fast forward to curtain up – what happens when you make love? In men, orgasm sends sperm-rich semen shooting into the vagina and towards the cervix at about 10 miles per hour giving the little fellas a good send off as they embark on their long and hazardous journey – God-speed boys, God-speed.

As we discovered earlier, a woman's climax could well play its part too, the wave-like contractions helping to pull the sperm deeper into the cervix. So you've both done your bit and are happily enjoying a post-orgasmic cuddle and you're wondering if you've just made a baby; that and if the rest of that chicken from yesterday is still in the fridge.

Inside your partner, millions of your sperm are beginning their quest to find an egg. Tragically though, the scene in there resembles the first 15 minutes of *Saving Private Ryan*. If it's not the acid in the vagina out to burn them alive, it's the cervical mucus which hauls them back like quicksand. Out of the millions who began the trip, only a few dozen will make it to the egg, the majority getting trapped, fried, lost or, one would imagine, just plain depressed at the scale of the task they have been asked to perform.

It's carnage in there.

Only the very best swimmers make it the 7 inches from the cervix through the uterus to the fallopian tubes, with the real athletes arriving in as little as 45 minutes and the knackered old war horses, no offence to the girl sperm, limping in up to 12 hours later. But no matter how long it takes them, what the sperm are all desperate to find on arrival is an egg. If they don't find what they are looking for immediately, all is not necessarily lost – the sperm can wait there in a resting stage for 12–24 hours. Conversation between the tense sperm must be quite awkward at this stage I'd imagine, but the line 'Do you come here often' must feature at some stage surely?

Once a sperm does meet an egg, it then has to find the energy for one final push to get inside the egg before any of the others do. The very instant one is successful the egg effectively clamps down a protective shield around itself so that no other sperm can get inside.

Now that the race is over, the real work can begin as the genetic material in the sperm combines with the genetic material in the egg to create a new cell that starts to divide rapidly.

Technically pregnancy begins when that bundle of new cells, known as a zygote, and then an embryo, travels the rest of the way down the fallopian tube and attaches itself to the wall of the womb and bang, you're going to be a Dad!

Finding out and keeping quiet

When you think about it, such is the gravity of discovering that you have actually made another person – created a member of the most complex and profound species on the entire planet – that it's a wonder the news isn't accompanied by the sound of heavenly trumpets, rather than the tinkle of wee onto plastic.

Pregnancy tests: now and then

The home pregnancy test is of course a standard piece of kit in the modern world. In fact so sophisticated are the latest models that they have done away with the blue line appearing – no, no, that was way too confusing. Nowadays you get tests that don't leave anything to chance and flash up the words 'pregnant' or 'not pregnant'. But that's not all: they also tell you how many weeks gone you are too. It's only a matter of time one thinks before the gizmo is launched that tells you from the get-go if your child is going to like marmite, follow your football team or get a tattoo.

The vast majority of home pregnancy tests work by detecting the hormone 'human chorionic gonadotrophin' (hCG), which is secreted by the placenta into both the bloodstream and into the urine after passing through the kidneys, right after a fertilised egg implants in the uterus. Most tests offer a percentage accuracy rate well into the high 90s.

It wasn't until the 1980s that pregnancy tests as we now know them started to appear. Before that there were some really quite disturbing methods of detecting if there was a little person knocking around. The ancient Egyptians were the first ones to focus in on urine as the best place to start looking. But mixing wee-wee with different grains to see if they germinated was where the smart thinking stopped mind you. The quacks of the Middle Ages kept on sniffing around urine too, but their idea was to mix it with wine or whatever alcohol was lying about the place. Whether they then knocked it back in one before bellowing, 'It's a girl!' history doesn't record.

It wasn't until a century ago, when scientists were uncovering the secret world of the hormone, that the modern pregnancy test really began to take shape. This milestone was bad news for baby rabbits though – the *méthode du jour* of detection to find out if a woman was pregnant was to inject a urine sample from her into a little fluffy bunny. The only drawback was that in 100% of cases the procedure meant that the bunny died. As if that wasn't bad enough the results themselves weren't even fucking accurate! Happily, this wretched method didn't catch on and by the late 1970s a woman could test her own urine at home. But my God what a palaver it was – mixing with various solutions in a range of test tubes was required – a kind of baby home brew kit. But the home test was here and pretty soon it had turned into what we recognise today and will almost certainly be the way you find out that you're a father-to-be.

And when you do, it will mean you are... fecund.

What a word. Not only does it mean that you're a working specimen when it comes to reproduction, but it also sounds suitably, but not overly, dirty. The moment your other half waves that positive pregnancy test under your nose – but hopefully not too close – you are officially one fecund dude.

Be ready for the emotional rollercoaster

Congratulations big boy. You're about to enter a world full of words you've never heard before, sights you've not seen before and emotions so new to you that they will knock you flat on your arse.

For many men, the very moment they discovered the news is indelibly marked in the consciousness forever, a kind of JFK moment without the bullets. Some are on the end of the phone; some are standing right there with their partner waiting for the test to do its thing; some no doubt find out by text or heavens above, on Twitter.

But no matter where or how you discover the news, you'll probably be hit by an emotional double whammy. Firstly, there's the pride, bucketfuls of male pride – hearing for the first time that you've managed to make your partner pregnant somehow feels like you have lived up to your highest potential as a man, that you are fit for purpose.

The second emotion that almost all the Dads I have spoken to admit to feeling is relief. Secretly, it seems, many of us fear that we are sterile right up until we get the ultimate confirmation that it's not blanks we're firing. Whether it's the unfeasibly tight pants we wore in our youth, the Marlboro Lights we used to suck on greedily as young men, or just a gloomy sense that those near misses in our past were wide of the mark because our sperm are sinkers rather than swimmers – many of us seem to have been harbouring a real sense that we would have severe problems getting the job done.

A survey carried out by American psychologist Jerrold Lee Shapiro in the 1980s [2] also claimed that once the shock and excitement of the news dies down, many men experience an irrational but very real fear that the child being carried by their partner is not theirs. After interviewing more than 200 men, Shapiro found that 60% of them held 'nagging doubts, or fleeting thoughts that they may not be the father'. Although only two of the men expressed genuine concern that their wives may have had an affair, the rest were 'expressing a general insecurity brought on by being part of something as monumental as the creation of life'. Either that or their particular partners were way too smart to get caught.

Finally, after dispelling the worry of sterility and banishing unfounded doubts of parentage, what has really happened finally starts to sink in during Month 1, and you begin to imagine how your friends and relatives are going to react to the big news.

Except you can't tell them.

That's right, the news that you've created the beginnings of a completely new life, a totally new person – the biggest thing you've had to tell anyone ever – you have to keep firmly tucked under your little hat.

Spreading the joy

If ever you wanted to tell someone something it's this. God knows we have enough bad news to impart over the course of our lives – so let's ring out the bells, take out a page in the paper and let everyone know how clever we are.

But that's not the way it works is it? Modern wisdom dictates that you don't spread the word until you reach the three-month mark and you've had a chance to check it actually is a baby. Imagine the embarrassment if you were to tell all and sundry that you were expecting early on, only to find out during the three-month scan that your partner's stomach pains were actually caused by a Sky+ remote.

So that's where it went.

The three-month silence is a far from universal or uniform practice though. Many people choose to tell parents or close friends, as much to gain early support in the tough first few weeks as the desire to spread the joy. There is no right or wrong way of doing it, just what suits you and the mother of your child best.

Around the world things differ somewhat too. In Java, pregnancy is announced right from the off and celebrated with ceremonial feasts and rejoicings – which sounds lovely doesn't it? Then again in several other cultures the whole thing is kept secret for a belt bursting seven months to avoid various superstitious ills.

So maybe we should just be grateful for what we've got.

Of course, there are sound reasons why the vast majority of people choose to keep quiet until the first trimester is out of the way – and almost all of them centre on miscarriage. As we are about to discover, almost 98% of miscarriages happen within the first 13 weeks of pregnancy, so it's easy to see why many couples choose to keep the news close to their chests.

....

Words from your fellow man:

Tom, 34, father of two: *We were in bed at my wife's sister's house and Jane said she thought she was late, had sore boobs and had been sick. Years of avid Colombo watching led me to conclude we needed to purchase a pregnancy test.*

The next day on the way to her parents we stopped off at Tesco Extra and Jane bought one there and then, leaving me to the shopping. With a knowing look from the till lady she headed straight to the toilets, past a security guard who had clearly seen it all before.

Meanwhile my shopping continued and I came across cans of Napolina chopped tomatoes on buy one get one free. As I loaded my 11th and 12th tins into the trolley, I saw Jane at the opposite end of the aisle. A smile, a nod, small tears of joy and we were expecting our first baby.

After a long embrace, the trolley was emptied of all tinned goods and I headed straight for the organic veg aisle.

Enzo, 36, father of one: *My wife bought me a book entitled* Conception, Pregnancy and Birth *in the hope that I would read between the lines and discover that she was pregnant.*

I didn't.

I simply focused on the word 'conception' and thought to myself 'here we go; she is going to get me to eat lentils for the next six months to boost my fertility...'. In the end, she had no choice but to show me the two positive test results and shout 'I AM PREGNANT'.

The M word

A fair chunk of your partner's time – and therefore your time – will be used worrying about miscarriage across the first months of pregnancy. The fretting and the nervousness is relatively unavoidable

I'm afraid and the sad fact is that miscarriage is not an uncommon occurrence.

The often-quoted figure is that around 20% of all pregnancies end in miscarriage, but this is increasingly being seen as a woefully conservative estimation. Many miscarriages can and do happen without women even realising they were pregnant, putting the episode down to a heavier than usual period.

With that taken into account, the miscarriage rate is thought to be more like 40% or 50% – with some experts going as far as to say that almost every sexually active woman will have one at some point in her life, whether she is aware of it or not.

Whatever the true figure is, what's for sure is that miscarriage lurks around the first three months of pregnancy like a menacing playground bully; probably never likely to strike, but always carrying a threat.

With that in mind it's worth getting clued up on the real facts and figures around miscarriage, rather than listening to some of the more widely held myths and scare stories – that way you can sleep a little easier, and, more importantly, you can help the mother of your child navigate through what are often choppy early waters.

Some of this doesn't make for particularly pleasant reading and if you want to skip on to happier pastures please feel free to do so, but knowing exactly what's going on, what to look out for and what to avoid could be crucial if you are unfortunate enough to experience the heartache of a miscarriage.

What is a miscarriage?

The word miscarriage itself refers to the loss of a developing pregnancy until the 20th week of gestation. Medical terminology, in all its clinical glory, labels this event a spontaneous abortion.

Not surprisingly, most women who miscarry would react pretty badly to hearing that phrase at such a traumatic time, but it is worth noting that 'abortion' merely means the loss of a pregnancy – it doesn't assume that the pregnancy ended out of choice.

There are three types of miscarriage:

> **Complete miscarriage:** This means that the woman's body expels all the tissue. Symptoms include the passage of all pregnancy tissue and a closed cervix.

> **Incomplete miscarriage:** This occurs when the body expels part of the pregnancy, with portions of the foetus, amniotic sac or placenta being retained. Symptoms can include cramping, and the discharge of blood and foetal matter.

> **Missed miscarriage:** This means that the woman's body doesn't get rid of the dead foetus itself. Missed miscarriages may go unnoticed for weeks and symptoms may include a lack of feeling pregnant. However, due to the high hormone levels, some women go through this awful experience even while experiencing a wide range of pregnancy symptoms.

Management of miscarriages that are missed or incomplete often includes dilation and curettage (usually referred to as a D&C). In this procedure, doctors manually open the cervix and get rid of what's inside the uterus.

What causes a miscarriage?

Although this is somewhat of a grey area, it seems pretty certain that foetuses that have some kind of abnormality tend to miscarry. For instance it's thought that around half of all first trimester miscarriages are the result of chromosomal abnormalities that prevent the foetus from developing as it should.

Another, similar, cause is that the foetus did not implant, or bury itself, into the womb lining properly – again, down to bad luck rather than carelessness or bad decision making either by your partner or yourself.

Maternal age can be a factor though. For women younger than 35, the miscarriage rate is 6.4%; for those aged 35–40 it is 14.7%; and for mothers-to-be over 40 it's 23.1%. A woman is also at a higher risk of miscarriage if she has had more than one miscarriage already [3].

Another area where there is thought to be a link is through the use of certain painkillers. A study carried out in the US in 2003 backed up findings from a Danish report two years earlier that taking ibuprofen or aspirin increases the chance of miscarriage by up to a massive 80% [4]. Although many authorities view these findings with caution and have called for much larger studies to confirm them, the results still cause many women to avoid aspirin and ibuprofen altogether and stick with paracetamol as their pregnancy painkiller of choice. There has been no link found whatsoever between paracetamol and miscarriage.

The warning signs

The most obvious signs are period-like pains and heavy bleeding, but your partner could miscarry without even knowing, especially very early in pregnancy.

The sight of blood during early pregnancy doesn't always signal a miscarriage. Often called spotting, light bleeding is fairly common and it's estimated that about 15%–25% of women experience some sort of bleeding in the first trimester. Although in many cases it turns out to be nothing, the medical advice is unanimous – at the first sight of bleeding during pregnancy, no matter how light, contact your doctor, midwife or hospital straightaway for advice, even if the bleeding eventually stops.

The aftermath

Losing a baby is a tragedy, no matter how early in pregnancy it takes place. Like almost every other emotional event in our lives, everyone's feelings vary. You and your partner may want to start trying to get pregnant again straightaway, or you may differ on that score. A degree of apprehension and anxiety at the thought of going for it again is almost unavoidable. Medically most doctors advise waiting until your partner has had at least one period before trying again, but emotionally it's much more difficult to put a generic timeframe on it.

The sense of loss you both feel may be similar or poles apart. It may also be linked with the type of miscarriage you had; later or missed miscarriage, which involve medical intervention, obviously causes a great deal more emotional and physical upheaval.

The knowledge that early miscarriages in particular could well be nature's way of stopping something that isn't quite right before it really starts, does sometimes help people to rationalise what has happened – and as men that kind of logic can give our brains the capacity to move on. No matter what the circumstances though, getting over a miscarriage, especially for the mother, is never to be underestimated.

But no matter how awful your experience may be, or how deep your sense of loss, take some heart in the fact that the vast majority of couples come together, help each other get over it in their own time and go on to have a happy and healthy baby.

Words from your fellow man:

Chris, 34, father of one: *Since we've had our first we've suffered two miscarriages. The first was because of a condition called trisomy 13 – the baby forms and is alive but its brain doesn't form as it should, there's no face, too many digits – it's horrific. Most die in the womb before birth, a few make it but die very shortly afterwards.*

We were gutted to say the least and it hit my wife particularly hard and she was in meltdown for a long time. We were told,

*however, that there was no lasting damage and that we could try
again. So we did.*

*This time we were soon told we had identical twins. I had a
good feeling about this one, but my wife was understandably
nervous as hell leading up to the three-month scan.*

*As a vet, she can pretty much 'read' the screen of the scan. I
can't. As I was staring at it trying to find the image of a baby,
my wife just looked at the doctor in terror – and he just said, 'I'm
sorry' – we'd lost them. Then all hell broke loose. Talk about raw
human emotion flooding out. We cried for days.*

Levi, 36, father of two: *When our first child was nearly two,
my wife had a miscarriage at about eight weeks. She bled heavily
for two weeks and felt very poorly. Her next period, maybe two
months later, was a mixed bag of emotions for her, she was sad
that it was definitely the end of the pregnancy, even though she
had rationalised it well up to then.*

*I was upset but without a doubt, my wife suffered more. But
it's something we could get through, and was not the end of our
world. I think the reason we managed it OK was through her
strength of character. We agreed we would try for a baby as soon
as she felt OK again. As it happens, it took a little longer than we
thought for her to get her head round things, but we managed to
conceive again about four months later.*

Ectopic pregnancies

While we're under this dark but necessary cloud, it's probably worth
getting ectopic pregnancies dealt with too. Given the relative rarity with
which they occur – it happens in about one in every 100 pregnancies
in the UK – this complication certainly punches above its weight in the
scare-the-shit-out-of-you stakes.

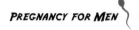

What is an ectopic pregnancy?

This condition is essentially a pregnancy that develops outside the womb (ectopic means 'in the wrong place'). It can occur in several places: the ovary, the abdomen, the cervix, at the join between the tube and the womb, all over the place, but by far the most common area is within the fallopian tube.

As the pregnancy grows, it causes pain and bleeding and, if not recognised, the tube can rupture, causing internal bleeding. It's not pretty and unless treated quickly, it can be fatal. No matter where it occurs and how it's treated, the pregnancy itself never makes it – it has to be completely removed.

Most commonly found between the fourth and tenth week of pregnancy, the most common reason for an ectopic pregnancy is thought to be a blockage or narrowing of the fallopian tube, which stops the egg from making its way to the womb. Instead, it implants where it can.

How to spot an ectopic pregnancy

Generally these nasty little buggers show themselves in two ways:

> A missed period and positive pregnancy test accompanied by some abdominal pain, quite often on one side, and some irregular bleeding. This is by far the most common way of discovering something is wrong.

> As a full-on medical emergency. Without warning the woman becomes deeply unwell, collapses and is taken to hospital. A positive pregnancy test is found and she is transferred to theatre there and then and a ruptured ectopic is found bleeding into the abdomen.

Now you can see why this particular complication has developed a very bad name for itself.

How is it treated?

In a small number of cases the ectopics will not rupture and will be naturally absorbed back into the body. Another small percentage of cases can be treated with a drug that makes the pregnancy shrink away by stopping the cells from dividing.

But the vast majority of instances will require either keyhole surgery or more traditional open surgery. Whichever of these routes is taken, two courses of action are open to the surgeon, either to open up the tube and remove the pregnancy, or remove the tube altogether.

Around 65% of all women who have an ectopic conceive again within 18 months [5], but for many other women, their fertility can be affected – and affected badly depending on the damage done to one or both of the tubes.

The aftermath

Given the drama and danger that goes with an ectopic pregnancy it can be easy to forget that as a couple you have also lost a very much wanted pregnancy and that just as with a miscarriage, the grieving process may well take time.

The progress report

Someone once said that a week was a long time in politics. It won't surprise you in the slightest to learn that (i) the person in question was himself a politician and (ii) that he was talking shit.

If you want to experience weeks where truly momentous things happen, things like growing a heart from scratch, or creating not one, but two eyes out of a bag of gunk, then the womb is the place for you. As well as the often blistering pace that your soon-to-be son or daughter sets when it comes to growing, your partner doesn't hang about either.

These little progress reports will give you a man-sized (by which of course I mean very small, and easy to understand) run down of everything you need to know about the changes the two most important people in your life are going through month by month.

The age of your baby

In order for us to take this information on board in palatable monthly chunks, rather than week by week (and I've not met a man yet who doesn't have to use his fingers, toes and teeth to do the endless converting from weeks to months throughout the entire pregnancy) we need to do a bit of nifty maths at this stage.

Your baby's age can be determined by counting the first day of your partner's last menstrual cycle as Day 1. Although she wasn't actually pregnant on that day, this is the system – the gestational age method – that most doctors use in determining due date and therefore how old your wee one actually is.

This means that we add in the extra two weeks (it can obviously be a few days either way, but 14 days is used as a standard measurement) that it takes to get back to the first day of the last period. See p 189 for more on due dates.

All that adds up to mean that Month 1 for the baby is counted as running from the first week to the sixth week. Don't worry if that has made your nose bleed, pretty much every other month is just your standard four weeks long, so Month 2 is from the seventh week to the 10th week and so on.

The progress report

Month 1 (Baby is 1-6 weeks old)

Your baby

Your little one is on fire. At the end of this month your baby will be about the size of a raisin; but what a raisin!

Once the fertilised egg is embedded in the lining of the uterus, it multiplies and grows at an astonishing rate. What was originally a sperm/egg combo is now officially a blastocyst (fluid-filled ball) comprising several hundred cells. Pretty soon though this blastocyst divides into two.

The half still attached to the womb will become the placenta – unlucky. The other half will become your baby – jackpot.

The baby section then divides into three layers which will go on to form your baby's body. The innermost layer will later develop into the thyroid gland, pancreas, lungs, liver, urinary tract and bladder. That's quite a layer you'll be thinking, but wait.

The middle layer will become the entire skeleton, all the muscles (including those in the heart), testes or ovaries, spleen, blood vessels, blood cells, kidneys and the dermis, the deepest layer of skin.

And the outer layer pulls its weight too – this will provide the hair, nails, tooth enamel, the lenses of the eyes, epidermis, sweat glands, and nipples.

By the end of the first month the beginnings of the spinal cord are in place and there's even a rudimentary, but very much beating, heart – and all this while your partner may well just be thinking that she has a bad case of wind, rather than a microscopic miracle taking place inside her.

Your partner

For most first-month mothers-to-be there is a distinct lack of symptoms. Your partner may feel slightly premenstrual – that's right, that old friend is still lurking around – and she may pass urine more often than usual or have sore breasts. Some women may even get the first knockings of morning sickness. But compared with later months the first handful of weeks is a veritable breeze for your good lady.

But that doesn't mean there isn't stuff happening to her. The hormone progesterone is busy making her cervical mucus thicker and more gloopy, eventually forming a plug. This, as the name suggests, is nature's way of putting a big, snotty bouncer on the door to stop anything getting in or out.

THE MUST-DOS OF THE MONTH

You'll love 'being pregnant' as you will now find yourself saying in an ever so slightly camp way. But don't let me give you the impression it's a doddle. Your partner is about to go through a series of physical and psychological changes of gargantuan proportions. What's more, you, yes you, will need to become her masseuse, her counsellor, her bag carrier and her punch bag – all while trying to get your own head around becoming a Dad.

It's far from easy, but to help you navigate your way through, here are three little things you can do this month that will make your partner happy and earn you bags of brownie points.

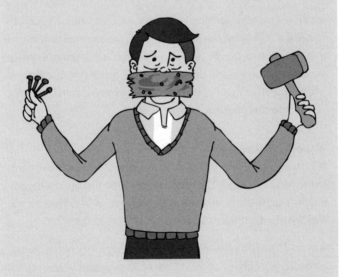

Mum's the word

Sounds simple this, but worth a mention for sure; if you've agreed with your partner not to tell anyone your big news until the three-month scan, for Christ's sake don't blurt it out to your mate, your mum or your boss. No news travels like pregnancy news and by the time you get in that evening a 30ft banner will adorn your house saying 'Nice One Gob-shite'.

Testing time

Make no mistake: your reaction to the positive pregnancy test result will be remembered, regurgitated and requoted for decades to come.

For the love of God don't let any fear or anxiety you may be feeling turn into words at that precise moment. If you're feeling like the contents of your stomach have divided equally and are heading to both your north and south orifices, keep it to yourself and tell her later after the initial moment has passed.

It's an overwhelming thing to find out that you are on your way to being a Dad and it has the potential to mess with your head for a second or two, but be positive and warm, she's probably twice as scared as you are and the last thing she needs is you screaming 'shiiiiiit'. Besides there's plenty of time to worry yourself sick later – just enjoy this moment.

A spot of bother

It's startling how easy it is to worry yourself into sheer blind panic once you're expecting. The urge to protect the tiny life is a trigger-happy little blighter and can, if you're not careful, lead to you making situations a whole lot worse rather than better.

A typical example of where a cool, calm head is needed, is vaginal bleeding, or spotting. Around 25% of all pregnant women suffer some sort of bleeding in the first trimester, with more than half of them going on to give birth to a healthy baby at full term.

Bleeding doesn't necessarily mean miscarriage; it doesn't necessarily mean anything is wrong at all in fact. In many cases it is down to breakthrough bleeding – the hormones that control the menstrual cycle can cause bleeding when your partner's period would have been due.

Another innocent explanation could be implantation bleeding – when the fertilised egg attaches itself to the wall of the uterus causing spots of blood to appear in your partner's knickers.

At this point, screeching 'Blood, blood, there's blood' isn't what's called for. Your partner will be petrified with fear as it is and your calm reassuring presence will work wonders.

If your partner does experience any level of bleeding whatsoever at any point in the pregnancy, the thing to do is call your midwife, doctor or hospital straightaway to get it checked out.

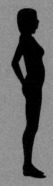

MONTH 2
Say hello to my little friend

For many women the first month of pregnancy is a bit of a non-event in terms of the physical impact it has on them. For a minority it's the first of many months of nausea.

All in all though, the tiny little bag of cells buried deep inside a woman's tummy doesn't really make its presence felt early. It quietly goes about its business, dividing and growing, growing and dividing, feathering its nest for the long journey ahead. But once it has got its newly formed feet under the table by around the second month, it often says 'Hello there', in a number of not-so-pleasant ways.

Let's tackle the little blighters one at a time shall we?

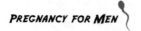
Morning sickness and co

Morning sickness

Morning sickenss is for the Ford Focus of pregnancy symptoms. Everyone's heard of it, lots of women have it and nobody likes it.

First things first, it doesn't just happen in the morning. Whoever named it patently got bored waiting around, witnessed a couple of morning chunders and thought 'Sod this, I'm off for lunch, that bad boy is hitherto called "morning sickness"'. Nausea and sickness can and do strike a pregnant woman at any time of the day, or even at night.

It's reckoned around eight out of 10 mothers-to-be feel sick at some point, with half of them actually vomiting. Symptoms vary wildly from woman to woman. The lucky ones will get the odd bout of mild queasiness, whereas others will be struck down by the severest, truly debilitating, form of the complaint. If your partner suffers from this, you are both in for a tough time. She will be vomiting morning, noon and night, unable to eat and drink properly, and even losing weight when she should be putting it on.

It's serious shit and many women who get chronic Nausea and Vomiting in Pregnancy (NVP), to call it by its clinical name, often feel like no one takes their plight seriously or understands the magnitude of what they are going through – which can lead to depression.

Why morning sickness occurs is a bit of a mystery. One theory is that the changes in hormone levels during the early stages of pregnancy may cause short-term nausea and vomiting. The pregnancy hormone human chorionic gonadotropin (hCG) is thought by many to be the culprit – which is why those women expecting twins often suffer from worse morning sickness because they are producing more hCG. Oestrogen levels also rocket during the first three months, coinciding with the time that morning sickness is at the peak of its puke-inducing powers. Rising levels of oestrogen may heighten the sense of smell too, which may explain why certain pongs can trigger the onset of symptoms.

The second predominant theory is that it's all Darwin's fault. Many scientists believe that NVP is an evolutionary adaptation to ward women away from eating dodgy food.

You'd have thought that some kind of pamphlet would have sufficed.

The theory goes that morning sickness often puts women off eating foods that can potentially become contaminated, such as meat, poultry and eggs, and nudges them towards preferring foods that have a low risk for transmitting infections.

It's certainly true that pregnant women have a sense of smell that would safely see them into a career as a police drugs dog. That tuna melt you had at lunch will start to soon see your bloodhound partner run screaming out of the back door the moment you walk in through the front. It's also been suggested that substances such as alcohol can set off a bout of sickness. NVP is nature's very own booze prevention officer; keeping new mothers-to-be off the sauce by making them spew their guts up at the mere mention of a white wine spritzer.

As with many facets of pregnancy there are also 101, let's say more *challenging,* theories as to the cause of morning sickness. My favourite is that it's the result of the mother-to-be's loathing of her partner; the subconscious manifestation of which is a desire to abort the foetus through vomiting. Take a bow Sigmund Freud for that belter.

One thing there is agreement on is that on the whole, morning sickness does no harm to the baby at all provided that the mother-to-be can keep some food and fluid down.

In fact, recent thinking sees morning sickness more as a sign of a healthy pregnancy, signifying that the female sex hormones which keep the placenta implanted in the womb are plentiful. But I seriously wouldn't try to float that cheery piece of news by your partner as you are holding her hair back for the 15th time that day. You might just find your suede shoes pay a hefty price for your misplaced positivity.

In most pregnant women, NVP starts to ease off between the third and fourth month mark, but for some it lasts longer and for a cursed few it stays with them for the entire pregnancy.

What can you do to help?

One thing you shouldn't do is try to insist that your partner continues to force down a healthy balanced diet if it makes her hurl. A spell of eating little else but grapes, Scotch eggs and the salt off Tuc crackers isn't the end of the world – and if that's all your partner can keep down then that's what's for dinner.

Luckily the mother-to-be's liver stores a lot of the nutrients the baby needs to keep on track, so a spot of weird eating doesn't do any damage (make sure she keeps taking a folic acid supplement though).

A few other tips that you might like to suggest are:

> Avoid drinks that are cold, tart, or sweet.

> Drink little and often, rather than in large amounts.

> Eat small, frequent meals that are high in carbohydrate and low in fat.

> 20 minutes before getting up, eat some plain biscuits. This one seems to get passed on from generation to generation and is, if nothing else, a good excuse to snack in bed.

> Avoid piping hot meals – clever one this. Cold food doesn't give off as much of a smell as hot food.

Sore boobs

Let's be honest, there are those among our gender who find it hard not to show appreciation for their partner's more curvy areas via the medium of touch. If you are one of life's well-meaning gropers it's important that you take this on board: during early pregnancy many women have extremely sensitive and sore breasts – keep off.

As their body gets ready for the months of pregnancy to come, they produce the hormones oestrogen and progesterone and it's these two blighters that are the main culprits behind what can be a pretty troublesome pregnancy symptom. As well as the hefty hormone surge, your partner's breasts are also beginning to store fat and increase in size as milk glands start to appear ready for the big feed once the nipper arrives.

The worst of the sore-boob phase has usually passed by the end of the third month, so despite the fact that they are almost taunting you by becoming even more fulsome and attractive, the least you can do is keep your hands to yourself for a while.

Hurting hooter

Before we move on from soreness, one pregnancy ailment that doesn't get much of a look-in but can cause nagging discomfort is something called rhinitis of pregnancy.

Our old friend oestrogen basically makes the inside of the nose swell and can even trigger the production of more snot – leading to a constant runny or stuffy nose for around 20%–30% of pregnant women. Nice.

Constipation

Women who suffer from chronic constipation during pregnancy are often truly plagued. Irregular bowel movements and sluggish, turgid, intestines can make their lives, well, shit really. And when constipation's side-kick from hell – haemorrhoids – pops up, or out as the case may be, then things really do turn nasty.

And who's behind this anal Armageddon? That's right; it's those dastardly hormones again. This time they are causing the muscles in the bowels to relax on the job. There is at least a decent reason for this particular disruption, the general go-slow means that food stays around longer so more nutrients are absorbed for both mother and baby.

All is not lost though, here's three key ways you can help your partner avoid a major log jam.

> Fibre is your best mate in the fight against constipation. Plenty of fresh fruit and vegetables, whole-grain cereals and breads, legumes and dried fruit, all help to get things moving. But for the sake of the neighbours don't let her jump right in to a fibre-rich diet if it's a departure from the norm – she will develop wind and bloating like you would not believe.

> Eating six mini-meals a day rather than three full-blown ones can make a significant difference.

> Water, fruit and vegetable juices not only get things moving, but soften the stool so when it does finally make an appearance it's not like passing a pine cone.

Exhaustion

Imagine – your body is hard at work on every level creating, housing and nourishing a new life. Your sleep patterns are shot to buggery because you're uncomfortable or restless or weeing every 35 seconds. You've spent half the day vomiting and the other half worrying about miscarriages. And, oh yeah, your fecking hormones are doing their bit to keep your bowels nice and clogged too.

Pregnant women get very, very, very tired. Even former dirty stop-outs who thought nothing of a 3am finish on a school night, soon fail to make it through *Eastenders*. The best way to cope is simple. Give in.

That sounds straightforward, but of course it isn't. If your partner loves her job or can't bare to miss out on what her friends are up to, she may well fight it for a while, but both work and social engagements eventually have to come second to the relentless waves of exhaustion that early pregnancy can bring.

You can help here in a big way by encouraging a reduction of her list of daily activities right down to the essentials, stocking the fridge with healthy ready meals, turning down the odd social do and making it possible for her to fit in a daily nap. Although it's different for everyone, the chances are that she will begin to feel like her old self during the second trimester, before coming to a grinding halt at about eight months.

It's also worth bearing in mind that once the baby is born you will be begging on hands and knees for just four hours of continuous sleep – so the pair of you should make hay and kip like nobody's business while still you can.

Heartburn

This is an all-too-common pregnancy complaint and can cause real and prolonged discomfort for the whole nine months.

Progesterone (yes, another trouble-making hormone) slows down the movement of the gastrointestinal tract which essentially causes food to just sit in the stomach. Not content with that, it also softens the oesophagus and lessens its pressure, which allows stomach acid to head north rather than staying in the depths where it bloody well belongs.

Get this though: the opening in the diaphragm that the oesophagus passes through from the chest into the abdomen can widen during pregnancy. This delightful scenario is for all intents and purposes a hiatal hernia, and if a portion of your partner's stomach slides up through this gap, it can cause havoc with stomach acid going back down. This type of heartburn is worse when lying flat so often strikes at night.

Obviously though most women who suffer from heartburn during pregnancy get a form that can be dealt with by using a normal antacid. The important tip here is to take the medicine about 15 minutes before your partner eats – otherwise she is just pouring it over the semi-digested food like some hellish whipped cream advert, rather than letting her stomach lining absorb it.

Mood swings

As we've seen, it's fair to say that pregnancy brings with it an eruption of hormonal activity on a volcanic scale. Almost every symptom, every change, is driven by a heady cocktail of chemicals – the word hormone itself means to 'spur on' and you can see why.

This potent pregnancy pina colada unsurprisingly also leads to mood swings and heightened emotions of all types for the mother-to-be. Of course this is all played out against a backdrop of the whole gambit of feelings that having a baby throws up too – joy, fear, worry, excitement – they are all there in spades, so pour on a canful of petrol of hectic hormones too and it's little wonder that the odd tear is shed.

And that's just by you.

Many women find that their moodiness flares up at around the (Month 2) mark, reduces in the second trimester, before reappearing to stir things up a bit ahead of labour.

Your role within all this is key. It's easy to find yourself fretting that you aren't reading the right books (although of course you are at the moment), buying the right kit (of which there is more on p 112) or generally worrying whether you will be able to cope. Although you may well be all at sea too, you are fortunate enough not to be drunk on hormones, so trying to instil an air of calm and confidence could well bring things down a notch or two.

Physically your partner's body is changing too and she may be starting to feel unattractive, or even that she is putting on too much weight. Again, keeping an eye out for these feelings and riding to the rescue with a few chosen words or a cuddle can work wonders.

Then of course there are arguments. Even though it's really, really hard at times to avoid a row with someone who is crying at the weather forecast one minute and screaming at a cupboard that refuses to open smoothly the next, the onus is on you to take one for the team, swallow the bitter pill of righteousness and end any rifts quickly. Think of the children man, think of the children. Good luck.

Words from your fellow man:

Colin, 33, father of one: *From about six to 15 weeks my wife was sick three to four times a day, every day, without fail. Everything from detergent to chewing gum set her off and she ended up having to take medication as she was getting really ill. Morning sickness has a bit of a jokey reputation, but when it's bad, it's a real curse.*

Levi, 36, father of two: *My wife has a tremendous sense of smell at the worst of times, but I would quite often be sent to the spare room if I had eaten something smelly or done something unspeakable in bed. Quite right too.*

While alcohol was out of the picture a new brew took its place in my wife's life – Gaviscon. She was getting through a bottle a day at the height of her habit. I was boozing for two at this stage, so we clung to each other for comfort like a crack fiend befriending a heroin addict.

There were also more tears at adverts than normal. Soap operas were often washed down with a good cry too.

But my wife remained calm throughout.

Only joking. She was a nightmare.

Once, on a long car journey when I was driving at 80mph down the motorway, she just said 'I have an overwhelming urge to hit you'. She managed to hold off, at that point anyway.

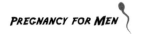

Suki, 34, father of two: *The fact that your partner's boobs become incredibly sore at the very same time that they look absolutely out of this world is conclusive proof that God has a fully functioning sense of humour. And is probably a woman.*

Sex and pregnancy

Now then. There's a fair bit of rubbish trotted out about what pregnancy does to a couple's sex life – the main lazy stereotype that masquerades as fact is that women get pregnant and completely go off sex – turning men into walking, talking gonads, driven to distraction and much worse, as they hump the nearest chair leg in a bid to sate their unfulfilled sexual needs. While that may happen to some, the picture is far more complex than the 1970s sitcom model of pestered wife and groping husband suggests.

Before we delve headlong into what really goes on when three-in-a-bed finally becomes a reality in your relationship – albeit not in quite the way you'd painted it in your filthy little mind – let's look at the facts around sex and pregnancy.

First things first. With a normal pregnancy having sex is safe right until your partner's waters break. Unless you have a traffic cone for a penis there is no way you can hit, prod, nudge or poke your baby. Surrounded by amniotic fluid, shielded by a drawbridge-like cervix and sealed by a mucus plug, your offspring is incredibly well protected and an ample but limited appendage like the one we all carry around with us just doesn't have what it takes to gatecrash the pregnancy party.

As we will see later though, those reassuring words count for absolutely nothing once you are actually in situ. There isn't a man alive who hasn't let the proximity of his angry penis to that of his tiny baby's soft little head cross his mind at the most inopportune of moments.

There's also no link whatsoever between having sex while pregnant and either early miscarriage or premature birth.

There are, though, certain circumstances that can make sex during pregnancy unsafe. Women who have any of these health complications should seek medical advice before doing the do:

> A previous premature birth

> Leaking amniotic fluid

> A history or high risk of miscarriage

> Unexplained vaginal bleeding, discharge or cramping

> Placenta praevia (a condition in which the placenta is low and covers the cervix)

> Incompetent cervix (when the cervix is weakened and opens too soon)

So if none of the above applies to your partner you are home and dry. Of course there are certain things you should avoid – inserting any objects into the vagina that could cause injury or infection for one, you dirty boy. If your sexual technique involves blowing air into your wife's vagina, not only do you need to seek professional help, you also need to avoid doing it too, because it can force a potentially fatal air bubble into her bloodstream. Nipple stimulation also needs to be removed from your repertoire, it releases the hormone oxytocin, which can cause contractions – and as we all know there's nothing like a contraction to put a dampener on things sexually.

But generally the message from the world of medicine is that as long as your partner is having a straightforward pregnancy and you're not a colossal pervert, you can have sex as much as you like.

But will either of you fancy it?

Feeling up for it?

After talking to many, many fathers about how their sex life was affected during pregnancy, it's clear that there is a wide range of scenarios that play out around sex, with different months heralding different feelings and libido levels for both partners.

But despite this fluctuation, for the majority of couples, a rough pattern does seems to emerge of how sex life changes through the pregnancy.

First trimester

The first trimester, with its vomiting, heartburn and constipation, funnily enough sees many women relegating sex to somewhere just below 'get toe nails pulled out' on their priority list. But plenty of men don't exactly feel rampant at this stage either, and the often-cited reason for a lowering of the libido is the Darwinian feeling that somehow the job has already been done.

As ever there are exceptions to this – more than a few men said that they enjoyed wilder, more passionate, sex with their partner in the first few months of pregnancy than they ever had before. Some said this was down to feeling a new closer bond with their partner, others that they were still testosterone fuelled after having their masculinity confirmed by the positive test result – and a few said that the freedom of not using contraception was what spurred them on to new pleasurable heights.

For the most part though, sex seems to be put on the backburner for the majority of couples during the early throws of pregnancy.

Second trimester

Once the fierce initial pregnancy symptoms die down for women, the second trimester can usher in some serious how's-your-father it seems.

This mid-way sauciness is down to more than just a lack of morning sickness though, our old friends the hormones can contrive to make women feel super-sexy and super-sensitive, with increased blood flow to the pelvic area meaning all sorts of receptors are switching on to woooooooahhhhh mode. So much so in fact that some women find the increased blood flow also increases their ability to have an orgasm or two, or three.

Add to this the increased voluptuousness, sexy curves and general glow that many women start to exhibit at this stage of proceedings and you've got one hot mama on your hands who you may well struggle to keep up with.

Of course for some women the exact opposite is true. Many find sex during pregnancy painful, others have huge self-image issues as their body changes and others even pay for their multi-orgasmic state by feeling abdominal cramps during or after they climax, which can even set off a wave of mini-contractions!

Third trimester

As the due date nears, sex can often fall away again as the now sizeable bump becomes a physical, and especially for many men a psychological, barrier to getting intimate.

Being kicked by your own child as you lie on top of its mother and have sex with her is perhaps one of the oddest things that can ever happen to you as a man. The notion of your penis being inches away from a living, breathing baby in itself has the power to dismantle an erection in seconds. Throw in the fact that your child can actually hear you grunting and groaning at this stage too and round it all off with actually seeing or feeling them move while you are at it – and it's easy to see why for some men the final trimester signals a real slow down in sexual desire.

Then of course there's the logistics of it all. A huge great tummy with a huge great baby in it does get in the way somewhat, so some lateral thinking on the position front is needed.

A survey of 3,000 new mums carried out by The Baby Website in 2008 [6] found that a whopping 58% said their partners had been scared of hurting them in bed, with half of the men wanting to stop sex altogether to ensure they didn't do any damage.

A similar poll [7] also found that 39% of women said the second trimester had definitely seen them have a sexual surge. However, the same survey also found that when given a list of options and asked, 'Which of these would you prefer?' although a relatively healthy 27% went for 'uninterrupted sex with your partner', 38% said 'a good night's sleep' – a choice you will come to understand and empathise with very soon. So it seems that how you and your partner deal with sex during pregnancy really has as much to do with your individual personalities and the state of your sex life before conception, as it does with any standard pregnancy horniness template that can be consulted.

What is relatively predictable though is that more than a few men are drawn into affairs while their partner is carrying their child. American psychologist Jerrold Lee Shapiro [8] believes that men who have these destructive dalliances share some surprising characteristics:

> They felt attracted to their partners and were very interested in affectionate or sexual contact with them.

> They felt particularly excluded from the pregnancy process.

> The affair they have is often with a close friend or relative of the woman.

The last point, says Shapiro, indicates that the person with whom the man has the affair also felt excluded from the pregnant woman's life. Either that, or the screwing couple are simply a pair of absolute shitbags.

Another pretty spurious reason that has been put forward for why men stray during pregnancy is that in their heads their partner has become off-limits sexually; a mother figure to be worshipped, not defiled with sexual acts. That is essentially like saying 'I adore and respect you so much now you're pregnant that I'm fucking a woman I met on the train instead.'

Infidelities aside, sex during pregnancy is pretty much a suck-it-and-see situation, if you see what I mean. You and your partner will find what works for you, which could mean experimenting with different positions, having the time of your lives during the second trimester, or ditching intercourse completely and focusing on less intrusive ways of getting intimate. Whatever you both decide to do, as long as you keep talking and touching you won't go far wrong – and never underestimate the power of a kiss and a cuddle.

Words from your fellow man:

Peter, 33, father of one: *It never really appealed to either of us, we were only going to give it a go for the novelty value. If I'm being honest I was pleased of the rest.*

Levi, 36, father of two: *Sex was infrequent throughout to say the least. It was useful towards the end when we found out at an antenatal class that there's something in sperm that can bring on labour. I had to fight hard to resist the temptation to ask the instructor if it could be taken orally mind you.*

Colin, 33, father of one: *Sex wasn't a massive issue, although we did try a few times – I'm not sure what it was but there was a physical and psychological barrier there for both of us. Oh yes, I remember, it was a baby.*

Jim, 34, father of one: *A friend had told me that he got loads of blow jobs from his partner during pregnancy. What a joker he turned out to be. To be honest the regularity stayed much the same and if anything it was a bit more romantic, a little more sensual. Once the bump arrived it became more sensual still, slower. Perhaps even lazy.*

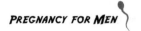

The progress report

Month 2 (Baby is 7-10 weeks old)

Your baby

By the end of this month, your baby will be four times the size it was at the start of it. That is quite a growth spurt, by anyone's standards. Having said that, even after expanding at such an indecent rate, the little fella is still about the length of a fun-sized Mars bar.

Your baby's head is also growing at an alarming rate to make way for its relatively gigantic brain. A neck is also beginning to develop and the primeval tail, which has momentarily developed down at the base of the spine, will be is reabsorbed back into the body. Probably for the best that.

All major organs develop in this intense period and the heart, although no bigger than a peppercorn, begins to beat strongly. Wrists and fingers begin to appear on the end of the still-forming arms, and legs start to develop with, amazingly, tiny little toes already appearing on the ends.

Under the baby's paper-thin skin its face starts to take shape too; bones fuse, the beginnings of a nose is formed and the outlines of the cheeks and a jaw can be seen. Inside his mouth sits a minute tongue.

Genitals have even begun to develop.

All this on a mini Mars bar.

It might be happening in thousands of wombs across the planet, but it is still an amazing feat of genetic engineering.

Your partner

As we've seen, for many women this is the month when junior and his hoard of hormonal henchmen announce his arrival on the scene in a big way.

As well as the symptoms outlined earlier, your wife's metabolic rate starts to increase and she will begin to take in more protein, more calories and often an inordinate amount of Rich Tea biscuits. All of this is fine and best not mentioned.

Although she won't look pregnant yet, her uterus has actually doubled in size since conception and that could result in a tighter waistband, which as we all know can bring with it a fair amount of upset in itself – so be prepared to lavish compliments from now on.

Finally, the blood supply to your partner's vagina and vulva increases in a big way from now on and they both tend to turn a purple colour. So please don't be alarmed.

THE MUST-DOS OF THE MONTH

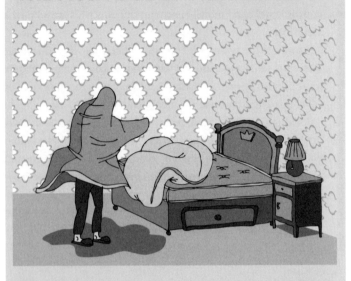

Tuck her in

Changing bed linen is a job with a very high pain-in-the-arse rating – every man knows that. Every man also knows just how much better you sleep on lovely, cool, new sheets. Chances are your partner is more exhausted right now than she has ever been in her life. You know what to do.

The cat's done a whoopsy

Cat crap can pose a very real danger to your pregnant partner. A horrid shit-inhabiting bug called *Toxoplasma gondii* lurks in cat faeces, as well as in unwashed fruit and veg. If caught by a pregnant woman it can be transferred from her via the placenta to her baby. The infection has the potential to cause miscarriage, blindness in the foetus or damage to its nervous system.

If you've got a cat, emptying the litter tray is your job now my old son.

Read the next chapter now

The three-month mark sees the first scan being done and all the joy, nerves and occasional heartache that can bring.

Knowing what's going on ahead of time will help reassure you and your partner so you know what to expect and not put yourselves through any undue worry.

She will also think you are the dog's bollocks of a father-to-be – which of course you are.

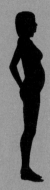

Month 3
Show and tell

I n a lot of ways this is one of the toughest months of all. Morning sickness and its outriders of early pregnancy misery are often in full swing; the fear of miscarriage hangs around like the smell of a damp dog on a blanket; and the time comes to do two joyful and simultaneously scary things.

First up we have what for most people is the first set of ultrasound scans. On one hand it's a time of almost overwhelming wonderment to be able to see your baby for the very first time – or a map of a particularly bad storm over the Orkneys depending on how good your sonographer is – but it's also a moment of worry. Lots and lots of worry.

Second, once you've negotiated that little emotional minefield it's time to break the peaceful pod you and your partner have been living in for the past 12 weeks and tell your news to the cruel, cruel world. Again for many it's a joyous time, for others a proper pain in the arse full of underwhelmed mates and overwhelmed family members, or vice versa.

So then, with your tube of gel at the ready, let's have a close look at what you'll be mainly watching this month. Your baby.

The early scans

It's worth saying before we kick off that the scanning of babies in the UK is not a uniform science. You'd think it would be, wouldn't you? You'd think there would be a nationwide plan that smoothly kicks into place and calmly tells you and your partner when, where and why you'll be having what.

Don't be daft. Like cancer care, bin collections, council tax and two-to-a-bed graveyard plots, it all depends on where you live. Things have improved enormously over the past few years, but it's still a hotchpotch, leaving some people having to fork out privately to have certain tests. Chances are though you will be in an area that gives you everything you need when you need it.

Ultrasound scans have been used in pregnancy for around 30 years now and have an exemplary safety record, with no side effects being found whatsoever. They work by sending high-frequency sound waves through the womb, which bounce off your baby before being turned into an image on a screen.

Hard tissues such as bone reflect the biggest echoes and show up white, with soft tissues coming out grey. Fluids, such as the amniotic fluid that your baby lies in, come up black as the echoes pass right through them.

Your sonographer will interpret these images, or failing that, guess. Apart from the gel being a little chilly on her tummy, the only real discomfort caused to your partner is down to the curious fact that to obtain a better picture she needs to have a full bladder while it takes place. Just what a wee-machine needs.

The dating scan

All pregnant women should be offered a dating scan when they are between 10 and 14 weeks pregnant. As the name suggests this is to primarily nail down exactly how pregnant your partner is in a bid to avoid her going full term in Sainsbury's when she actually thinks she still has a month to go. Also, because hormones vary at different stages of pregnancy, pinning down exactly what stage she is at is vital for future tests to be valid.

That isn't all the scan does though, it can check that your baby has a regular heartbeat and is developing normally – which is always nice to know, isn't it? Your baby's head, hands, feet and limbs can all be seen after a fashion and even some organs can be viewed. Depending on the quality of the equipment any major limb abnormalities can be picked up at this stage but the main major news you could find out is that you are expecting twins, triplets or more.

If you have recently discovered that you are expecting a multiple birth, put this book down immediately you lunatic. You've got no time for reading my good fellow – you should be out there hunting for that crucial third job, or at least just be asleep in a vain attempt to bank some glorious shut eye before you effectively cease being human and become a milk-mixing machine.

Alright, it might not be quite that bad, but man alive it must be the test of all tests. Although they are on the increase, thanks to higher instances of *in vitro* fertilisation (IVF) treatment, multiple births are still rarer than you might imagine; out of 764,000 births in the UK in 2007, only 11,500 were twins, with just 149 triplets, three sets of quadruplets and one set of quintuplets being born.

Listen to the beat

There's a good chance that this scan will be the first chance you get to actually hear your baby's heartbeat, as well see it on screen.

If you're lucky and the sonographer or midwife can find it using the hand-held instrument, you'll hear a noise that resembles someone bouncing a basketball in a wind tunnel – a frighteningly quick boom, boom, boom accompanied by a shed load of crackling and white noise.

What will really amaze you though is how strong your little one's heartbeat sounds – it's hard to imagine a more resounding confirmation that there's a separate life taking shape than the thumping and relentless pound of a baby's heart in its mother's tummy.

The picture

There's something iconic, almost Warholesque about traditional baby scan pictures. The moody shade and light, the somehow comfortingly shaky detail, the tantalising first ever glimpse of a new life.

There are new kids on the pictorial block available – three- and four-dimension scans that you can fork out for from the month five mark to have your baby turned into something resembling Jabber the Hut covered in caramel.

Now, if ever you get more for less (and I say less rather than nothing because even the standard images will now set you back a few quid a pop), it's in the field of the baby scan. Pull out the garish confectionary 4D close-up from your wallet at work and you're likely to have to calm a few people down. Get out a good old, fuzzy, ultrasound image and you'll have a queue of folk desperate to have a gander and lie through their teeth to you about being able to see the head – 'and look, look, there are the toes.' There's something very reassuring about that.

The scan of my son Stanley is on the heaving notice board above me as I write this, and looking back, his perfect little profile really did give us a peak at how beautiful he would be; just as your baby will be too. The only thing misleading about it, is that he looked like he was asleep, which we now know would have been highly unlikely.

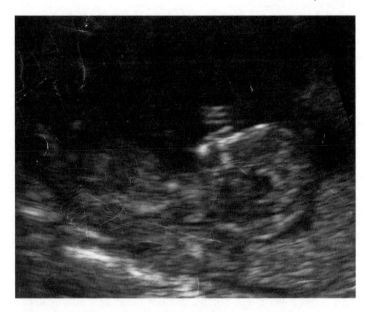

The Classic Scan. Yet more snow forecast for the Grampians

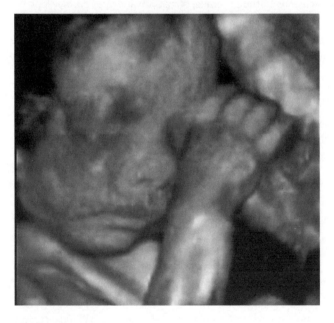

Buddha takes a nap

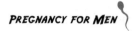

The nuchal translucency scan

This scan isn't half as much fun.

Nuchal translucency (NT) is the name given to a build-up of fluid under the back of a baby's neck. All babies have some of this fluid, but many babies with Down's syndrome have an enlarged amount.

To be effective the scan must be performed between 11 weeks and 14 weeks and almost always happens at the same time as the dating scan – any earlier than this and it's too hard to perform, any later and the excess fluid can be absorbed by the baby. Many hospitals offer an NT scan to all women between these dates but it isn't available everywhere, and you may want to have it done privately.

Using ultrasound, the NT scan measures this area of the neck and the results give a likelihood, but crucially not a definitive diagnosis, of a baby having Down's. The image is often poor, and the way of measuring on the screen is startlingly crude, but as you and your partner look on with a strange feeling in your stomach, time stands still. The results of this, your child's first ever test, could have a profound effect on all of your lives.

To calculate the risk the sonographer enters the measurement together with the other crucial piece of information, such as your partner's age, (the risk moves from one in 910 at age 30 to one in 28 at age 45), into a database and you are given a risk factor of your baby having Down's there and then.

No matter what the meeting, no matter what your boss will say, you can't miss this scan. Finding out news like this, even if it's good news, isn't something a pregnant woman should do alone – although of course many do just that.

If the results show your pregnancy as low risk, as the majority are, then you hug, kiss and move on to the next milestone. If they put you in a high-risk bracket – one in 150 or less – you have some crushingly difficult choices to make. Combining an NT scan with a blood test gives a more accurate result, raising the detection rate from around 75% with the NT scan alone to around 90%. You'll be very lucky indeed though to find this test, called the combined test, on the NHS. While this combined test isn't available on the NHS everywhere, it is steadily becoming more widespread in England. If you're in Scotland this isn't the case so you may still have to go private.

If this scan finds you are high risk, the only way to know for certain if your baby has Down's is to have a diagnostic test such as chorionic villus sampling (CVS) or amniocentesis, both of which come with the risk of miscarriage, with between one and two women in every hundred thought to lose the baby because of the procedure. CVS is believed to carry the slightly higher risk.

Both procedures are invasive, meaning that they use matter collected from the placenta in the case of CVS and fluid from the womb for amniocentesis. Choosing to have either of the procedures is a fantastically complex and emotional decision, and of course in the relatively unlikely event that the information you get back from them is the news you fear, you face the ultimate gut-wrenching choice.

....

Words from your fellow man:

Chris, 34, father of one: *I was pretty nervous at the three-month scan stage. My wife is very medically minded being a veterinarian, so was the researcher from hell in terms of what could go wrong – glass is half empty – whereas I am a glass half full merchant, so I just assume by default that everything will be alright.*

The Down's syndrome scan was my first indication that there are actually a multitude of things that can go wrong and often do. It also started discussions about the 'what ifs' which makes you question some very big moral values as a couple.

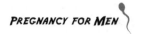

Enzo, 36, father of one: *We failed the general screening and decided to go with one of the two invasive Down's syndrome detection tests.*

In some cases, the chances of miscarriage being provoked by one of the invasive Down's tests such as the CVS are appreciably greater than having a Down's baby. This makes the decision to proceed with such tests very difficult indeed.

Spreading the word

By the time the choppy waters leading up to the first scans have been navigated through, some couples are bursting at the seams to tell all and sundry their news; one of them almost literally.

Many others though have come to love the little bubble they have constructed around themselves. Despite the vomit, the heartburn, the moodiness, the tears (and of course whatever the mother-to-be may have been through too), they have become a real unit, the two of them and their tiny little baby. And now they've got to spoil it all by saying something stupid like 'I'm pregnant'.

Of course you've got no choice; pretty soon your partner will give the game away in a quite spectacular abdominal fashion and besides, telling everyone often turns out to be a fantastic time and means you and especially your partner can talk about what you're going through with other people who've been there.

If they don't already know, parents are usually first on the list, and depending on your circumstances their reaction can range from hyperventilating joy and the immediate drawing up of a list of things to buy, through to cardiac arrest and the immediate re-drawing of wills. Hopefully though both your folks and your in-laws will be nicely placed nearer the shopping list end.

If your child represents the first grandchild for either set of parents there is also the chance you'll come across the 'I don't want to be called

Grandma' reaction, which while initially upsetting and unsettling, will almost certainly melt away when your beautiful baby holds Grandma in his tractor beam gaze.

Siblings can fall into different camps as well. Brothers and especially brothers-in-law who already have kids, often display a very distinctive look among the generally congratulatory noises they make. This enigmatic facial cocktail can only be described as two parts glee (that your boozing, holidaying and restauranting days are about to be curtailed too) and one part resigned sadness (that another one has bitten the dust), all topped up with the soda water of genuine happiness that you will soon be experiencing the unmitigated brilliance of being a Dad.

Then there are your mates.

The difference between telling Dads and non-Dads is immediately obvious, the first batch are wearily interested, in the way that they are wearily interested in most things these days; and the other lot couldn't give a toss and besides will probably be out getting pissed anyway so won't get your text for two days. The bastards.

It's much trickier telling other couples though. Look out for a muted response at best, or full blown melt-down at worst from couples who unbeknown to you have been trying to conceive for two years.

Your partner's single female friends will pretty much follow the pattern you'd expect. The ones that have always liked you hope you'll repay their faith by doing right by their now pregnant and vulnerable pal. The ones who've always thought you a complete fuckwit will start to imagine how they will swoop to the rescue when the inevitable happens and you finally admit to being gay; probably just as the contractions kick in.

A more hackneyed set of stereotypes you'll be hard pushed to find, but as with all typecasting you are almost certain to come across at least one of the blighters when you break the news.

Crucially, if more mundanely, your partner doesn't need to tell her employers about the news until 15 weeks out from the big day – so for God's sake make sure she doesn't let it slip. A boss with early warning of maternity leave can be a very dangerous thing.

Chances are though any nerves you may have about telling the world will be washed away by tears, cheers and if you're very lucky, a few beers.

....

Words from your fellow man:

Donald, 34, father of two: *We used the most foolproof broadcasting method there is when we wanted to get the news of our pregnancy out there – we told my sister.*

Tom, 34, father of two: *We decided to tell close family only, until the three-month scan was out of the way. Unfortunately for my wife though, any lack of drinking was deemed so completely and utterly out of character that people were guessing left, right and centre.*

The progress report

Month 3 (Baby is 11-14 weeks old)

Your baby

By the end of this month your baby is fully formed. Job done, the show's over, move along, nothing more to see here.

Well not quite. All he needs to do now is grow. Not that he's been hanging around on that front for the past four weeks either – length-wise he's gone from a mini Mars bar to pretty much the full-blown version. That's a lot of work, very little rest and next to no play at all.

All of your baby's major organs have formed and his intestines have even been packed away neatly in his abdomen. He has nails on his toes and fingers and could even have some hair.

The little champ has even started drinking. Not being able to get out much, it's more of a quiet one at home swallowing amniotic fluid and weeing it out like a good 'un. Inside his miniature little mouth there are even tooth buds.

There's some serious movement going on now as well – knee jerks, back twists and the odd all-body hiccup – not that your partner will be able to feel any of that yet. Oh, and your baby can also smile, frown and suck his thumb if he is so inclined.

All of this awesome development means that from now on your baby will be at less risk because the critical phase of growth has passed. You can breathe a little easier from now on.

Your partner

For most women these are the final few weeks of morning sickness and a range of other frankly rather annoying early pregnancy symptoms.

From now on though, as your baby and his entourage of support systems begin to expand at a greater rate, your partner will too. As well as the to-be-expected expanding waistline, it will also see her making even more trips to the loo than before, if that's possible.

It's also safe to come out of the cupboard under the stairs too: hormone levels will start to settle down from now on and that coupled with less worry about miscarriage means that the atmosphere in your household could well change for the better.

A trivial but welcome little bedtime bonus for you is that if your partner has had pre-pregnancy ice block hands and feet of a night-time, you'll miraculously find them nice and toastie from now on in. To help lower blood pressure to cope with the extra strain being caused by the baby, your partner's arteries and veins relax, warming up the extremities.

THE MUST-DOS OF THE MONTH

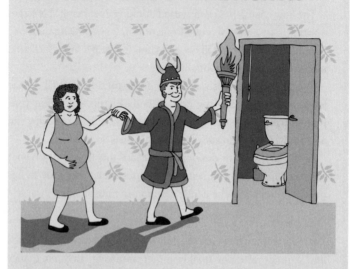

The light of my wife

There's going to be a lot of late night weeing going on in your house from now on. Put a small light in the path of your partner's route to the loo so she can see where she is going. Sweeping the route before you go to bed for any dangerous items she might trip over is a good idea too.

Take her away from it all

The beginning of this month can be a brute for your partner; little or no let-up in symptoms, scans on the horizon and six more months to go. Booking a night away in a quiet hotel will go down a treat, or if money is tight, a candle-lit night in with you waiting on her hand and foot before making time to talk about any worries she might have, will be long remembered.

Class act

This one is a blinder. Not only is it a very good idea, but I swear to you, if you do this, you'll be in clover.

Antenatal classes might seem a long way off in the seventh month or so, but the best ones get booked up way ahead of time. The sessions run by the National Childbirth Trust (NCT) get snapped up especially quick and have – rightly or wrongly – more of a reputation for forging long-lasting friendships among parents than some of the NHS-run ones.

Get online, get on the phone, find out the details and watch the mother-to-be of your child melt in admiration as you tell her you've been doing a bit of research into parenting classes.

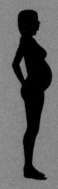

MONTH 4
I see you baby

We are but simple beasts, us men; we see it, we believe it. For many of us the moment we see our child on the scan screen, or hold the fuzzy but precious picture in our hands, is when we truly believe.

I'm not for one moment suggesting of course that until this point we suspect our pregnant partners of fabricating violent bouts of sickness, molten lava-like heartburn and a bladder of quite extraordinary weakness; we know she has a baby in there – but there's nothing quite like seeing it for yourself, is there?

This moment of tangible proof together with the start of the second trimester and its more physical signs of motherhood, can have quite an effect on a new father-to-be. In many cases it cranks up the level of interest in both the mother-to-be and baby to new, dizzying heights – which while generally welcomed, can, if not tempered, become as one medical professional put it, a right ball ache for your partner.

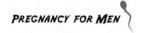

Of course you're not going to constantly question your partner about everything she eats, how much exercise she is or isn't taking, or whether she uses the mobile too much. You're a sensitive and well-balanced individual who will keep his concerns and fears in check, while trusting his partner's judgement implicitly. Just to be on the safe side though, here's a quick list of pregnancy dos and don'ts for you to have in your pocket, should your overactive worry gland get the better of you.

What's safe and what's not

Food and drink

The big one. From people at work helpfully enquiring 'Should you be eating that?' of your partner, to your well-intentioned mother saying that in her day raw egg was seen as a superfood, there's a fairly bewildering array of advice to be had on what is and isn't safe to eat as a pregnant woman.

Here's a rundown that should help clear up a few common worries, or alternatively turn you into a food Nazi.

> Oily fish is good for both mother-to-be and the developing baby, but there is a risk of high levels of pollutants, especially mercury. It's best to have no more than two portions a week of the likes of mackerel, trout and sardines, so all the benefits are reaped without chancing overexposure to any nasties. The old cupboard staple of tuna should be limited to no more than four medium-size cans or two tuna steaks a week. Swordfish, marlin and shark should be off the menu altogether – both eating them and swimming with them.

> Pâté is a no-no I'm afraid, no matter what it's made from or where it's been made.

> Blue cheese or types that are soft mould-ripened, such as Brie or Camembert, are out. Unpasteurised soft cheeses, such as those made from sheep and goat's milk should also be consigned to a 'The first thing I'm going to have when it's out' list.

> As well as being vile, raw or uncooked eggs are off limits. Supermarket salad dressings and most everyday mayonnaise brands are made from pasteurised egg and are safe though. Hurray.

> Unpasteurised milk and any dairy products made with unpasteurised milk can lead to food poisoning, meaning they should be history for nine months too.

> Eating meat is fine, but make sure it's well cooked with no pink or red bits. Should Britain ever have a summer to speak of again, take special care when eating barbequed food. Cured meat products, such as salami, are also best avoided.

Alcohol

Mmmm, alcohol and pregnancy. The advice on this seems to change on a daily basis but what's for sure is that no one really knows what a safe level of alcohol consumption is for a pregnant woman. The most comprehensively safe course of action is for your partner to go on the wagon either for the whole thing or for the first three months when your baby is doing most of its developing.

If giving up booze completely for the entire duration is just too much to bear for her, then the advice is to stick at no more than one or two units of alcohol, no more than once or twice a week.

You won't be surprised to hear that binge drinking is out. You may be surprised to hear though that a binge is often classed as having five or more drinks in a two-hour session. Yeah, worried now aren't you, booze boy?

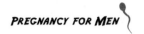

Exercise and pregnancy

You'd imagine being pregnant is as good a reason as anyone is ever going to get not to have to do any exercise. I'm afraid not.

Exercising in the right way during pregnancy is a very good idea indeed. Not only does it build muscle tone, strength and stamina (all of which can help your partner's body cope with the weight gained during pregnancy), keeping active can also make it easier to regain pre-pregnancy fitness levels after the birth and can even help to reduce constipation and tiredness, as well as circulation problems.

Of course, taking up hammer throwing or kick boxing wouldn't be the brightest move, but following a fairly straightforward list of dos and don'ts should see your partner get all the benefit without any of the risk that exercise, if done in the wrong way, can pose to a pregnant woman.

If you can help her to remember the following, she won't go far wrong:

> Exercise doesn't have to be strenuous to be beneficial – that walk to the shops counts too. As long as it's not the chip shop.

> The appropriate level of exercise will depend on how fit your partner was before she became pregnant. Tragically your semen has not turned her into an Olympic athlete.

> She should drink plenty of fluids when exercising.

> It's also wise to take a gentle approach to exercise that doesn't put strain on her joints and ligaments.

> Exercising during pregnancy isn't about losing weight.

> She shouldn't exercise flat on her back, particularly after 16 weeks, because her bump presses on the big blood vessels, which isn't a good idea at all.

> Don't use saunas or steam rooms, they make you too hot, and could poach your baby.

It almost goes without saying, but not quite, that any activity that puts your partner at risk of falling has got to be in serious doubt during pregnancy too. That doesn't just mean the obvious ones such as skiing and tightrope walking either; tennis and cycling for instance have to be done with extreme caution, especially as your partner's sense of balance may be more than a bit wonky thanks to the bowling ball she is carrying around with her.

Scuba diving and other sports that run the risk of planting a potentially deadly air bubble in her blood stream are out too. Walking and swimming seem to be the favourite choices of a lot of mothers-to-be, with pregnancy yoga coming up on the rails.

Is it safe to fly during pregnancy?

In the first and second trimesters, pretty much yes. The third trimester is out because not even the most accommodating of flight attendants wants to deliver a baby using a plastic spoon and the whistle from a lifejacket. Besides, wedging a woman in her ninth month into a plane seat isn't good for anyone concerned.

Be warned too, ticket agents don't tend to ask if you're pregnant when you book your seats, the little blighters, but there's every chance your partner could be questioned about her due date as she waddles up to the gate – and airlines are well within their rights to bar you from travel if they think there's a chance your partner might ruin the upholstery.

To confirm it's safe for you to fly it's smart to get written permission from your doctor if you can. If your pregnancy is complicated by medical problems you would do well to check with your GP before travelling at any stage.

Flying during pregnancy can slightly increase your partner's risk of thrombosis, but wearing support stockings will help keep her circulation flowing. Pregnant women should also give small planes that don't have pressurised cabins a miss too. As well as the air pressure issue, small planes (in my slightly panicky experience) are almost always shit scary and wobble around like a 1950s washing machine. Don't do it.

Hair colour

Hair colour! Yes hair colour. It might not seem like a big deal to you, but what seems like thousands of online message boards hum with the white hot chat of whether dying your hair is bad for your baby. Annoyingly no one has enough information to say with absolute cast iron certainty that using a lovely rusty red or mahogany brown during pregnancy is completely and utterly safe.

Animal studies have been carried out over the years, and some, but by no means all, have shown a handful of the chemical compounds in hair dyes to cause birth defects. In most cases though the animals were given doses way, way beyond what women would be exposed to.

With all this unsatisfactory information about, there's no wonder this issue always turns up like a bad penny – but the consensus at the moment is that if the dyes are applied safely, using gloves in a well-ventilated room, and not leaving solutions on for any great length of time, it probably is safe.

For some people though that just isn't good enough and many women use alternative routes such as highlighting their hair or using vegetable dyes such as henna while they are expecting.

Is it ok to wax during pregnancy?

As hair growth tends to increase for some women during pregnancy, this is another one that comes up more than you'd imagine.

There's no evidence to show that waxing is unsafe during pregnancy and if, like I did, you are wondering if the baby feels an agonising shock as the strips are removed – apparently they don't, so rest easy. Your partner on the other hand could well be in for a rougher ride than usual because her skin may become even more sensitive in pregnancy.

Is it safe to have dental work during pregnancy?

Not only is it safe, there's two very good reasons why your partner should go and see the dentist while they are pregnant.

Firstly, the hormones cascading through your partner's body can wreak havoc with her gums, and, secondly in the UK, dental care is free, free I tell you, right from the moment when pregnancy is confirmed, through to the little one's first birthday. That makes this the single solitary time where having a baby might actually save you some money, rather than emptying your bank account quicker than a credit card cloning conman. Root canal, anyone?

Is it safe to paint during pregnancy?

No one really knows. There's no doubt that painting does expose you to some pretty hefty chemicals, but because it's next to impossible to measure how much the body absorbs, calculating the risks is equally as tricky.

There is some evidence though that exposure to the type of chemical solvents found in paint does increase the chances of birth defects [9]. The study found that the risk of having a baby born with gastroschisis (a nasty and potentially fatal abnormality where the baby's intestines protrude through a hole in its abdomen) was up to four times higher.

There are guidelines for those women who do chose to paint, such as limiting the amount of time you spend doing it, keeping the windows open and wearing long garments to protect the skin; but by far the simplest and safest answer is for your partner to let someone else do the painting. That means you by the way.

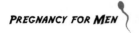

Are mobile phones safe to use during pregnancy?

Are mobile phones safe to use full stop? Who knows.

There has to be a chance, no matter how slim, that in 50 years' time when the first people to have had a phone stuck to the side of their heads for their entire lives start to reach their dotage, we may just start to realise that placing an electronic device next to your brain for long periods of the day isn't the smartest thing we've ever done as a species. Having said that current research suggests that there is no risk whatsoever to health from mobile phones in the short term.

If you're especially worried about your partner's mobile usage during pregnancy though, a good tip is that unbeknown to the majority of us, every single mobile phone is rated according to the levels of electromagnetic radiation that it emits. The SAR (specific absorption rate) value reflects the maximum amount of energy which can be absorbed by your body when you're using the phone. The higher your phone's SAR, the more radiation you are absorbing.

You'll usually be able to find the SAR rating of your partner's mobile in its instruction booklet, or, if like the rest of us, she threw that away without so much as glancing at it, stick 'SAR values' into a search engine and you'll find websites that will tell you the SAR of every handset on the market, as well as a whole load of scary information you'll probably wish you'd not read.

I'm suffering too you know

The concept of the phantom pregnancy, of hairy-arsed blokes clutching their backs or feeling a bit sick in support of their heavily laden but perfectly calm wives, is a comedy staple.

Only two of the multitude of new fathers I spoke to in the writing of this book were brave or stupid enough to admit to having shadowed any of their partner's symptoms.

It's easy to see why the whole idea is met with such ridicule. When researchers at St George's University, London, carried out a study [10] of 282 fathers-to-be in 2007, one of the men who admitted to being affected by the phenomenon came out with this little gem: 'I was constantly hungry all the time and had an unstoppable craving for chicken kormas and poppadoms. Even in the early hours of the morning I would get up and prepare myself one. It was strange to say the least.' By that definition I have been suffering from secondary pregnancy symptoms for the whole of my adult life.

Yes indeed, there's no wonder that the phantom pregnancy is viewed as a load of old twaddle put forward by bedwetting blokes who can't stand to be out of the limelight for nine minutes let alone nine months. Which is a shame, because recent research is beginning to paint a very different picture.

Couvade syndrome, as this phenomenon has been coined (it's from the French word meaning 'to hatch') has been documented throughout the ages and some studies put the number of expectant Dads who suffer from it in some shape or form as high as 65%. The condition presents itself in men with symptoms such as nausea, vomiting, stomach pain, back pain, toothache and exhaustion. For many the symptoms are pretty subtle, a spot of weight gain here, an unexplained ache or pain there. Other men though have full-blown mirror pregnancies, having exactly the same symptoms at exactly the same time as their wives.

So what, they're all mad, I hear you cry in your most uncaring and sceptical voice. But wait, oh cynical one, two heavy duty, bone fide studies carried out in Canada have found what may well be a genuine physiological rather than crackpot psychological cause for these symptoms: hormones.

Yes, those pesky hormones, the same buggers that make your partner's life a misery during pregnancy, can also give you a damn good going over too.

The two studies, conducted at Memorial University and Queens University in Canada [11], took blood samples from couples at different stages of pregnancy, as well as shortly after birth and monitored specific hormones because of their links to nurturing behaviour.

First up there's cortisol, which is seen as a good indicator of a mother's attachment to her baby. New Mums who are found to have high cortisol levels can detect their own infant by odour more successfully than those with lower levels for instance. The tests found that in expectant fathers, cortisol was twice as high in the three weeks before birth than earlier in the pregnancy.

Then there's prolactin, which among other things has been shown to bring on parental behaviour in a number of birds and mammals. The studies discovered that prolactin levels rise too, by around 20%, in men during the weeks before their partner gives birth.

That's not all either; the clever Canadians also discovered that fathers-to-be had elevated levels of oestrogen of all things, many weeks before and after birth. Best known as a female sex hormone, oestrogen exists in small quantities in men, too and animal studies show that it can turn males into super-sensitive fathers.

Then there's the biggy – testosterone. When sweet little birdies who have just become Dads are given testosterone, rather than looking after their new offspring, they strut around defending their territory and even mate with other females, the dirty birds. In humans, research has shown that males experience a surge in the levels of this hormone when they win sporting events and other competitions. It's probably fair to say then that testosterone isn't conducive to producing the most caring Dad the world has ever seen.

Guess what? The Canadian studies found that testosterone levels dropped by a third in new Dads during the first three weeks after the baby arrived. So essentially mother (or father) nature has found a way to engineer it so that the chemical that makes you such a chest-beating, arse-pinching fool of a man, reduces dramatically just at the very time that you need to bond and coo over your newborn baby.

So... what's going on?

There's a clue in that the Canadian studies mentioned in the previous section also found that hormonal changes in men closely parallel those of their pregnant partners. Although far from a scientific certainty, the smart money among the eggheads is that intimate contact and communication between partners is what brings on these changes.

In other words, spending time with a mother-to-be turns you into a father-to-be. Not in a psychological, 'Look at me, look at me, my waters have just broken too', kind of way, but in a very real physiological way. The same chemical forces that make your partner throw up for three months are essentially at work turning you into a more caring Dad.

Well I'll be buggered, as my own father is fond of saying.

Exactly how this hormonal osmosis takes place isn't known, but the transmission of pheromones looks to be a very likely candidate. Pheromones are potent chemical wafts that us animals constantly give off through our skin or sweat to stimulate other animals – usually in the 'I'm feeling horny' sense of the word. It's believed that pubic hair aides the transmission of pheromones, which is why we have kept hold of our underarm and pubic furriness while losing the rest of our body hair.

If women living in close proximity can synchronise their menstrual cycles via pheromones, as has been proved, then it's really not that

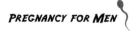

inconceivable that a pregnant woman lying next to her partner in bed could send a few chemical cocktails which start the process of turning him into a doting Dad. This intimacy effect, and the hormonal alterations it may cause, could also be the reason why many men experience pregnancy-like symptoms too. So as well as the umbilical cord attached to the baby, your pregnant partner also has an invisible, but powerful, link with you too.

Perhaps the best way to view this strange phenomenon though isn't that us men are being held in some sort of hormonal hypnosis by our pregnant partners, but rather that with a little help from them, nurture really is part of our nature.

It's still not enough to blame wanting a curry on though.

....

Words from your fellow man:

Jim, 34, father of one: *I definitely showed signs of a sympathetic pregnancy. I had headaches during the first few months and became exhausted on doing the slightest thing. That has continued after the birth too, but that's probably more to do with being actually knackered all the time than any phantom response. I also had dreams of having a baby, physically. Not sure if that is phantom or just weird.*

David, 34, father of one: *I've always thought this is a load of rubbish cooked up by blokes to try and get out of doing stuff – but felt seriously sick for the second and third months. I've no idea what else it could have been.*

The progress report

Month 4 (Baby is 15–18 weeks old)

Your baby

Be warned, your baby can now hear what you are saying. Fair enough, it might not be able to be able to make any sense out of which profanity you just launched towards the wobbly cyclist at the traffic lights, but thanks to its hardening inner ear bones, the little fella has begun to pick up its first sounds – which at this stage are mainly your partner's soothing heartbeat, rumbling digestion and all-important voice.

Despite still being only around 14cm in length and weighing in at not much more than 190g by the end of this month, complex pieces of kit, such as taste buds are already starting to develop. Crucially, lung development is steaming ahead too. Your baby is essentially doing breathing exercises, ready for the big moment when he will take his first breath once the umbilical cord has been cut. As these exercises happen your little one's chest rises and falls as his lungs begin to exhale amniotic fluid. Not to be left behind, the tiny heart is now capable of pumping as much as 24 litres of blood a day too.

Your baby is also going nuts on the workout front, twisting, turning, wriggling, punching, kicking and generally seeing what his amazing new body is capable of within the confined space he finds himself in.

You'll also be pleased to know that your baby's eyes aren't miles apart anymore either, which is nice.

Your partner

All things being equal your partner should be over the worst of her sickness and exhaustion and may well be feeling, if not full of beans, at least able to eat them.

Although your partner may not have gained a whole load of weight yet, in other, less conspicuous areas, her pregnancy really is motoring along now. Her nipples are darkening in colour (although you probably don't need me to tell you that), and down the centre of her abdomen she may well be developing a dark line, called the linea nigra, as the growing baby pushes her uterus out of its normal home in the pelvic area.

Her heart is now working twice as hard as it was before she conceived, with 6 litres of blood per minute being pumped around her body to feed the long list of vital organs that are being pressed into action to keep your baby growing.

Given the baby's gymnastics there's a good chance that towards the end of this month your partner (but not you) will be able to feel the baby moving for the first time – not the thumping great kicks that will boot you out of the bed in months to come, but a fluttering sensation that's been likened to having a flock of butterflies flying around in your stomach, or alternatively, wind.

THE MUST-DOS OF THE MONTH

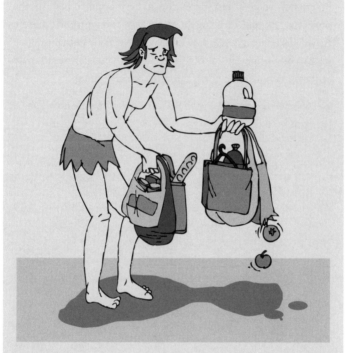

Me Tarzan

During the second and third trimesters the slightest fall for your partner can lead to some pretty serious problems. It sounds obvious, but gently suggest that you are now the chief lifter and mover in the household.

Dear diary

As the baby starts to move it's not a bad idea for your partner to keep a rough record of what she feels when. Buying her a journal that she can use to do just that is a good move and once baby is born she can use it to keep a track of feeds, sleeps, poos and, crucially, who has done the early shift most times each week.

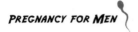
And relax

Pregnancy yoga is fast becoming a very popular part of the pregnancy routine for many mums-to-be – and with good reason. As well as being a gentle way to relax as her body goes through a myriad of changes, it's also a great way for your partner to meet other women who are going through the same thing.

Get yourself online and research a few courses in your area – she'll love you for it.

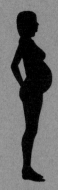

MONTH 5
Scans, flans and holiday plans

For some reason 'five months pregnant' sounds a lot closer to 'nine months pregnant' than 'four months pregnant' does, if you see what I mean?

Although you are still basking gloriously in the mid-trimester sunshine, with all its non-nausea and even a spot of sex to pass the time too, within the wonderful world of pregnancy there's something to worry about just around the corner.

In this case it's the anomaly scan, a brutally named ultrasound check to see if everything is as it should be with your rapidly developing baby. With a long list of deformities and complaints to search for, this is another squeaky bum moment on your journey to fatherhood, but as ever the nervousness comes hand in sweaty hand with the wonderment of seeing your, now very baby-like baby, up on screen and even, should you so desire, finding out if it's a boy or a girl.

Once what is almost certainly your last big scan before the birth is behind you, many couples take advantage of the mid-pregnancy lull and go on what will be their last ever holiday as a childless couple. Given the delicate nature of your partner's physical state, these little before-the-baby-breaks aren't always totally devoid of stress, but in general they are a fantastic, not-to-be-missed chance to spend some time together before all hell breaks loose. In a nice way of course.

I wouldn't want you to get the impression though that this month represents time off for your partner, a kind of commercial break in the middle of her personal pregnancy soap opera. Far from it. Just when she is giving a two fingered farewell to the symptoms of early pregnancy, another bunch ride into town, including the crazy world of cravings and the onset of what researchers believe to be the shrinking of the brain in all pregnant women.

The anomaly scan

Although it only takes around 20 minutes to perform, this scan covers an awful lot of ground. Most sonographers begin by showing you and your partner the baby's heartbeat and quickly pointing out parts of the tiny body before getting down to the serious business.

If at this point the screen is turned away from you, don't panic like I did, it's standard practice in many hospitals. The baby's head is often examined first, with shape and structure thoroughly checked. Although thankfully rare, many severe brain problems can be visible at this stage as well as the presence of a cleft lip, but not cleft palates which are hard to see.

Next up, your baby's spine is looked at to ensure that all the bones are in the right place and that the entire area is covered in skin. The heart is then given its MOT, with size and valve movement under scrutiny, the stomach gets a once over too, as do the kidneys. If your baby's bladder happens to be empty, the chances are it should fill up during the scan as it downs another gulp of that scrumptious amniotic fluid.

The position of the placenta is then checked to ensure it's not low-lying, a condition called placenta praevia, and the umbilical cord will also be looked at; the final box to be ticked is that the little mite has enough fluid to comfortably move around in.

Now the tape measure comes out, or at least an onscreen version, and your baby's head circumference and diameter are measured, as well as the size of his abdominal area and length of the thigh bone, bringing the nuts and bolts of the scan to an end.

This exhaustive list of checks can highlight about half of all major problems that could be lurking at this stage of pregnancy – remember though, we are talking about rare problems here. The Royal College of Obstetricians and Gynaecologists helpfully and somewhat scarily lists the chances of these abnormalities being picked up during this scan, should they be present, as:

> ❯ Spina bifida (open spinal cord): 90%

> ❯ Anencephaly (absence of the top of the head): 99%

> ❯ Hydrocephalus (excess fluid within the brain): 60%

> ❯ Major heart problems (defects of chambers, valves or vessels): 25%

> ❯ Diaphragmatic hernia (hole in the muscle separating chest and abdomen): 60%

> ❯ Exomphalos/gastroschisis (defects of the abdominal wall): 90%

> ❯ Major kidney problems: 85%

> ❯ Major limb abnormalities: 90%

> ❯ Down's syndrome (babies with Down's may have visible heart or bowel problems): 40%

Not a nice list.

If a problem is discovered, and again the chances are that none will, you'll be told straightaway. You should be given an appointment for a scan with a fetal medicine specialist within three days. A repeat scan doesn't necessarily mean the worst though. Most problems that need repeat scanning are not serious. About 15% of scans will be done again and most reasons are not found to lead to complications.

If though the second scan does indeed reveal a serious problem, you'll be given support to guide you through all the options and choices, none of which of course are easy.

Hamburger or turtle?

As with all scans, everything will go swimmingly for the vast majority of couples and the biggest dilemma they will face is whether to find out if they are having a boy or a girl.

While it's true that some health authorities don't give you the option because of fears over 'wrong gender' terminations, most will, and the 20-week scan is predominantly the time when people choose to find out.

Not that it's a cut and dried case of 'Where's the winkle?' for the sonographer, you understand – oh no, they can and do get it wrong. There are scores of stories of people being told they are expecting a boy, only to be handed what is quite obviously a little girl a few months later.

The problem is that even by Month 5, the boy bits and the girl bits don't look all that different. They are still very much a work in progress and when you throw in some dodgy old NHS equipment, a stubborn foetus that point blank refuses to open its legs and a sonographer who was a forklift truck operator 18 months ago, you can see why nailing the gender is far from a gimmie.

But bearing that in mind, if you and your partner are desperate to crack open the powder blue emulsion or hang those delicious pink curtains, there's a fair chance you'll be able to leave the 20-week scan daydreaming of playing footie with your boy, or telling your daughter that there's absolutely no chance that she is going out dressed like that.

An experienced sonographer will be on the lookout for one of two signs if you ask them to tell you the sex of your baby. In a girl the three lines that make up the clitoris surrounded by the labia are often charmingly referred to as the hamburger sign. In a boy it's the turtle sign they are watching out for, where the tip of the penis just peeks out from the testicles. It could just as well have been called the walnut whip.

Rather than putting your faith in modern medicine you can of course indulge in a spot of homespun gender detective work. There are countless ways of determining what you are having, with every country seemingly having its own methods. Here's just a selection of the most scientifically robust ones:

You're more likely to be having a boy if...

> Your partner's right breast is bigger than her left

> Your partner's pillow faces north when she sleeps

> Your partner is asked to show her hands and she presents them palms down

> Your partner's age at conception combined with the number of the month in which she conceived results in an even number.

You're more likely to be having a girl if...

> The exact opposite to the complete load of bollocks above happens.

Words from your fellow man:

Nick, 35, father of two: *They go very quiet in between taking measurements, which is understandable I suppose given they are concentrating so hard, but you end up waiting for a noise or listening to their breathing for clues. The thing that stood out was that after the scan it became apparent that this was the last time they were going to check on the baby until the birth – which felt as though we were going freestyle – alone for a long time.*

Chris, 34, father of one: *Before our daughter came along, I like many just assumed it's all a natural and straightforward process where the majority sail through easily. As it happens there's always something dramatic around the corner, or at least the threat of it.*

Levi, 36, father of two: *I was amazed by the virtual check-up the baby had at the 20-week stage. It's a real MOT before they are even born and I was stunned by what the scanner could see on screen.*

The babymoon

Travelling is never the same once your child arrives – and by travelling I mean anything that involves going out of the front door. Travel cots, baths, nappies, sterilisers, the dreaded baby bag and more toys than you ever knew existed, will turn a weekend away into a military operation with the potential to claim a casualty or two, namely your back and good humour.

Across the land Dads can be seen packing and unpacking cars like demented worker bees and if you watch carefully you'll notice that once they have expertly jammed the boot to its absolute capacity, the realisation dawns that they have left the 3-tonne pushchair/pram/travel system combo unit on the pavement.

Cue much bad language at best and a full scale breakdown right there on the street at worst. Not pretty. And that's just for three days in Devon.

For those brave enough to contemplate flying, packing the motor is just the beginning. The mumbling and grumbling of other passengers on the flight as your beloved tot starts to kick off is bad enough, but two hours in when the first 10 rows have got a petition together to hand to the pilot, you will dream of being somewhere, anywhere, else.

By all accounts things get easier as your family gets older and can be readily bribed with DVD players, but for the foreseeable future the wanderlust you once had will be put on the backburner; on the spare gas ring next to your friends, lazy Saturday morning breakfasts and any semblance of a savings account.

Bearing all that in mind, getting away in the second trimester if you possibly can is a smart idea on all sorts of fronts. With the risk of miscarriage and the bouts of sickness of the early months now hopefully in the past – and the third trimester a no-no for soon to be very obvious abdominal reasons – the second trimester holiday has become something of a well-trodden path in recent years.

Where not to go

While many women may experience an energy burst in mid-pregnancy, this quite obviously doesn't represent a green light to climb a mountain or book yourselves into that knife-throwing residential weekend you've heard so many good things about.

If you do venture overseas, try to avoid anywhere with a huge time difference and if ever your partner deserved a comfy bed and a fluffy towel rather than a backpackers' hostel, it's now.

The level of hygiene of your destination is also a key factor. Many vaccines are off limits and in the case of areas with a high risk of malaria, pregnant women need to think very hard before they travel, as they are especially vulnerable to the killer disease. Pregnancy makes women more susceptible to malaria infection and increases the risk of illness, severe anaemia and even death. For the unborn child, maternal malaria increases the risk of spontaneous abortion, stillbirth, premature delivery and low birth weight. It's not to be messed with.

Exposure to the sun obviously needs to be carefully controlled too – and not just for the obvious reasons. Some pregnant woman are particularly susceptible to a skin condition called melasma, otherwise known as (to be said in throaty film trailer voice) the mask of pregnancy. Melasma, which causes patches on the face, is believed to be connected to the female sex hormones oestrogen and progesterone – hence the link to pregnancy, and is made worse by exposure to the sun.

Those few factors aside, the world is, as someone once very nearly said, your lobster.

No surprises please

For many couples, the mid-pregnancy break lingers in the memory for years and can take on a real second honeymoon air as you take some time out to enjoy each other's company and talk about the momentous changes that are about to happen to you both. With the stresses and strains of labour and the early days of being parents just around the corner, it is time fabulously well spent.

For the love of God though, don't try to book it as a surprise. Despite her current mild-mannered appearance, your partner is still a pregnant woman and as such the chances of you taking every one of her many, many worries, fears and random thoughts into account and correctly choosing a destination are infinitesimally small. But bless you for thinking of it.

Earth, wind and forgetfulness

It really is quite staggering what carrying a baby can do to a woman's body and her mind doesn't get off scot-free either of course.

After the early raft of symptoms have hopefully all but subsided, another band of shysters often appear to take their place. While admittedly they tend not to be as unremittingly awful as vomiting every single day for three months, these new pretenders are worth knowing about because each of them has the potential to have a big impact on your partner and therefore you too.

Cravings

When a recent survey asked more than 2,000 women if they craved a certain food stuff or taste while they were expecting, more than 75% said they had [12]. That's a lot of women eating a lot of cheese flan with ice cream. What's more, half a century ago the figure was at about 30%. So what's going on? In short, no one really has a clue.

In recent years the notion that craving something represented your body crying out for whatever vitamin or mineral that particular foodstuff was rich in, really took hold and has been quoted by some pretty eminent pregnancy experts. A craving for chocolate for instance is put down to a shortage of B vitamins and red meat cravers were secretly in need of a protein boost. Currently though that nice neat explanation has taken something of a scientific kicking and given our culture's seemingly inexorable march towards mass obesity, it's not hard to see why.

If the 'cravings tell you what you need' theory holds water, as our bloated and enormous frames consumed more and more utter crap, Captain craving should kick in at some stage and send us sprinting to the nearest greengrocers to smash down the doors and devour every green vegetable we can get our hands on.

So, with that theory losing ground, what is responsible for cravings and the desire for odd flavour combinations in pregnant women?

The hormonal upheaval brought on by pregnancy definitely has the power to turn what was once a despised item into an adored one – and vice versa – and the need for strange textures has been cited as being behind why a lot of mothers-to-be crave ice. But no one really knows what's behind the phenomenon in truth, which makes dealing with it a bit tricky.

For most women their particular craving causes no real health problems, other than the psychological trauma of being stared at by fellow shoppers as she puts 98 courgettes on to the check-out at Sainsbury's.

Things can start to get serious if a condition called pica raises its head though. Named after the magpie, because of the bird's tendency to consume some pretty horrible stuff, pica is an eating disorder that causes craving for non-food items such as coal, earth, soap, washing powder, hair and cigarette butts. Mmm, think I'll cook for myself tonight.

The causes of this strange condition are pretty woolly too, but what's certain is that it can affect pregnant women and that emptying the ashtray into your mouth isn't recommended. If your partner develops a taste for Persil non-bio, gently suggest that she talks to the midwife or health visitor about it sharpish – and then put her on a spin setting.

Aside from the peculiar world of pica though, most food-based cravings are harmless and if it's what she wants, she's the one carrying the bowling ball around in her stomach so it's her call.

....

Words from your fellow man:

Peter, 33, father of one: *My wife decided to forgo prawns, blue cheese and white wine – and of course all three immediately became obsessions – but she held out. Nothing bizarre was eaten, but mountains of chocolate and cakes were consumed. Her pregnancy lipstick seemed to be a permanent dark shade of galaxy brown.*

Nick, 35, father of two: *Scotch eggs and cereal were the big winners on our weekly shop as my wife went through a lot of both – although thankfully not at the same time.*

Chris, 34, father of one: *My wife didn't have cravings, rather a complete aversion to pretty much all food, except for yoghurt, fruit and a white, it had to be white, buttered, it had to be butter, roll for lunch.*

Levi, 36, father of two: *Gin and tonic was the (largely) unrequited craving of choice for my wife.*

Wind

There's no easy way to tell you this, but your partner will almost certainly pass more wind from both ends during her pregnancy than you hitherto dreamed possible. The reason for this often sudden increase in gas, as our American brethren are wont to call it, isn't because she can no longer be bothered to pretend she's saintly in that direction, it's actually down to two separate little wind-generating factors.

Firstly, the hormone progesterone, which surges around your partner during pregnancy, relaxes the smooth muscle tissue throughout her body – which sounds lovely doesn't it? Unfortunately it also includes her gastrointestinal tract in this smoothing out process, which slows down digestion and generates bloating and lots and lots of wind.

Secondly, round about Month 5, as the baby slowly starts to crowd your partner's insides, her digestive system takes another pounding as it gets squeezed and manoeuvred about something rotten, leading to even slower digestion and an even higher food-to-fart ratio. Oh dear.

Helping her to reduce this troublesome gas, which can bring with it painful cramps, isn't all that easy. Part of the problem is that a lot of the foods that she has quite likely taken to eating to improve her diet are the biggest culprits of all. The old classics such as beans, brussels sprouts, broccoli, cabbage and cauliflower all contain a fantastically named substance called raffinose, which is pretty much as near to fart juice as you are ever likely to get. Then there are certain starches, such as pasta and potatoes, that can bring on a bout of belching and worse too, not to mention fibre-rich foods such as oat bran and a fair few fruits that can also stoke things up.

So if totally avoiding the foods that cause wind is all but out, what else can be done to stem the flow? Eating several small meals a day rather than one or two feasts is a good start, as is avoiding eating or drinking while scrunched up or lying on the couch. Other than that it's selective deafness and more tea vicar for you from now on.

Baby brain

Forgetfulness in pregnancy has been around for an awfully long time, but has only relatively recently made tentative steps towards becoming a bona fide, fully recognised symptom.

While it's nothing for either of you to get too worried about, it can be irritating at best, and downright disturbing at worst, for your partner to feel a few of her marbles gently rolling under the couch and out of sight – albeit temporarily. For the vast swathes of women who work through at least some of the time they are expecting, forgetfulness can be a real embarrassment with its potential to turn sharp minds into absent ones.

Over the past 10 years a number of studies have begun to suggest that 'mumnesia' as it's been called, is a nailed-on pregnancy symptom, allowing scores of women to relax about the fact that after putting the car keys in the washing machine they struggled for a full 15 minutes to remember their own husband's name to ask if he'd seen them.

Firstly, a study carried out at the Royal Postgraduate Medical School in London [13] found that the brains of pregnant women seemed to shrink during pregnancy. The researchers, who had taken magnetic resonance scans of mothers-to-be, found that the brain reduces noticeably in size during the pregnancy before returning to normal up to six months later. While the team responsible believed that the brain alteration was more likely to be caused by individual brain cells changing rather than the actual number of them decreasing, it's still quite a finding – albeit one that has been challenged in some quarters.

Secondly, more recently, scientists at Boston University and the Massachusetts Institute of Technology [14] have identified four driving forces behind the mumnesia phenomenon.

To start with there's a huge shift in priorities toward nurturing and looking after the little one. Who cares if your partner can't remember where she put her purse when she has got a tiny life to sustain? It's also worth taking into account – especially once the baby arrives – that you, the man of the house, very soon fall into the same category as the whereabouts of house keys – not that important in the grand scheme of things. Don't take it personally (yes you will), it's just nature ensuring that your partner is focused on the job in hand and not sorting you out or finding your cufflinks.

Our old friends the hormones also have a hand in things according to the study. Having rocketed early on, oestrogen levels, which, as well as playing a pivotal role in fertility also help to send signals to the brain, drop like a stone in the later stages of pregnancy and early motherhood.

Then there's the small matter of the pain of childbirth. The New England boffins proposed that the onset of memory loss could well be part of a cunning master plan to ensure that the horrors of the delivery room gently fade into the mists of time, meaning that sex is back on the menu, more babies are born and the species survives. Proof, if any further evidence were really needed, that God isn't just a man, Mother Nature is a cross-dresser too.

Finally the study calls on a cast iron banker to close the deal – fatigue. As well as the poor-quality kip that most women get as their pregnancy moves into its final stages, it's thought that the parent who takes primary care of a newborn loses up to 700 hours of sleep during the first year of its noisy little life. 700 hours! I forget what my legs do for a living after one night of less than perfect shut eye, never mind losing a month's worth of the precious, precious substance.

So all in all, it seems quite an historical injustice that pregnant women have been smiled at smugly for all these years as they hang their coat up on the fridge. In reality it's a surprise they remember to have the baby itself.

It's a contentious area this though and just as this book was going to print up popped another piece of research this time in the *British Journal of Psychiatry* no less [15], which said that after studying 1,241 women it had, finally once and for all, totally dispelled the myth of baby brain. So basically your guess as to whether this phenomenon actually exists is as good as the next university of scientists.

And if your partner's brain really does turn to mush, what can you do to help? As suggested earlier, you can buy her a little notebook that she can jot reminders down in. You can designate a special little spot in the house where car keys and other everyday items can live from now on. You can even remind her if she gets frustrated with herself that mumnesia is a proper pregnancy symptom like all the others and run through the reasons why, like the fountain of all pregnancy knowledge that you are rapidly becoming. But by far, the most useful tip to help her out while she is somewhat befuddled is to ensure that you never ever phone her while she's ironing.

The progress report

Month 5 (Baby is 19-22 weeks old)

Your baby

After weeks of relentless growth, once your baby reaches the five-month stage and is roughly 19cm long, his rate of expansion reduces somewhat (although his weight gain doesn't) and he focuses on other crucial areas of his development – like growing brain cells.

At the centre of his new little brain an area called the germinal matrix is busy manufacturing cells at an almighty rate. The production line stops before birth, but your baby's brain will keep on expanding until around the age of five years.

As nerve fibres get connected up and muscles get switched on like Christmas tree lights, your baby embarks on an ever-more elaborate gymnastics programme designed to improve motor skills and strengthen bones.

A thick white greasy substance, not unlike cottage cheese, is starting to cover your baby's body. Called vernix, it acts as a waterproof barrier to prevent his skin from becoming waterlogged in the sea of amniotic fluid he finds himself floating in. If only he had a stick of celery or carrot baton in there he could have himself his first ever snack too. Alas.

Down at the sex organ department, things are coming along very nicely too. If you're having a daughter her ovaries will already contain about seven million eggs, which will reduce to about two million at birth. In boys, primitive sperm have already formed in the testes ready for the whole process to start again in years to come. If he wants kids that is. No pressure, son.

A little welcome gift of baby's first ever turd is also progressing beautifully, as a delightful tar-like substance called meconium accumulates in his bowels.

Your partner

The single biggest thing that this month represents for the majority of women is the high water mark of wellness in the pregnancy. Your partner should be not too sick, not too sore and not too big, but just right – a healthy and glowing mother-to-be in her prime. If you're really lucky, all this good health will also mean she is feeling a little frisky and the increased blood flow to the pelvic area together with highly sensitive breasts, makes achieving orgasm more likely. For her that is, not you.

Of course, although your partner may be feeling as well as she has for a good long while, there's still plenty of tough stuff going on too as she moves ever closer to the big day. As well as the cravings, chronic wind and mushy brain, your partner's gums may well become spongy too and she is probably sweating more heavily than usual as her thyroid gland becomes more active.

Unfeasibly early as it sounds, your partner's breasts may also have begun to leak colostrum as well, the substance that will constitute your baby's first meal should it take to the boob.

But despite the farting, sweating, leaky breasted picture this chapter has painted somewhat, your partner is almost certainly looking unfeasibly beautiful at the moment.

Go on, give her a kiss.

THE MUST-DOS OF THE MONTH

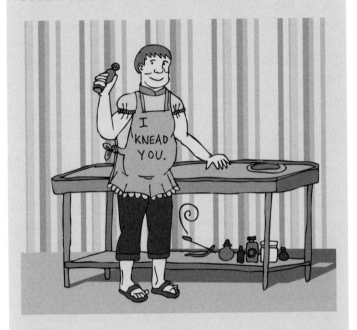

Magic hands

A spot of smart forward planning. In the coming weeks, various parts of your partner's body are going to ache, creak, lumber and throb like never before as the strain of carrying round a small person in her abdomen starts to really crank up. Be warned, you will be called upon, on a regular basis, to massage said body.

If, like most of us, your idea of a massage is 15 seconds of Chinese burn followed by a few karate chops, it might be a good idea to either do some internet research on a few gentle but effective massage techniques or sign yourself up to a quick course to learn the basics.

Dirty cash

As the half-way mark of the pregnancy is reached it's not uncommon for many men to be struck down with a severe dose of the 'How are we going to afford this?' flu. It's a nasty affliction which often strikes at night, rendering the bowels permanently open.

If you find yourself suffering from this, don't panic.

Many a bloke has pushed for a promotion, or taken on more responsibility in his job at this point, just to get a few more bob coming in. A year down the line though time will be the resource you crave the most, so stay cool, read the section in the next chapter on buying kit for the new arrival and rest assured that given the choice of seeing your face in the evening or having a cot that turns into an all-in-one printer at the push of a button, your baby and its Mum would much rather have the former.

Eau my God

The vast majority of us are dehydrated according to research. Drinking enough water is something almost everyone in almost every developed country is spectacularly piss poor at. While this is bad news for us all, as a pregnant woman it's to be addressed straightaway as water helps to carry nutrients to the baby and also helps to prevent infections, constipation and the dreaded piles.

To help your partner drink the three pints of fluid she needs (coffee, tea and pop don't count I'm afraid as they make you wee more out than they put in), make up jugs of water with wedges of lemon or lime in to help her overcome water boredom. If she hits you with the old 'But I'm suffering from water retention' line, sweetly remind her that the more water she drinks, the less her body will retain.

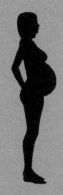

MONTH 6
Move over Dad

There's more of the pregnancy behind you at this stage than there is still to come. Scary isn't it?

It probably doesn't feel much more than half an hour ago that you had a plastic stick covered in urine waved in front of your face and the whole thing began. Since then you and your partner have almost certainly already been through two scans, a handful of scares and hundreds of night-time wees and morning time hurls. You'll have cried, laughed and argued in hopefully relatively equal measure and the excitement, together with a dash of apprehension, will be starting to build in a big way now.

Although you've seen the baby on screen and he has made his presence very much felt via his gang of hormonal heavies, the chances are the introduction of a fledgling third person in your relationship has so far pulled you and your partner closer together rather than making you feel less of a unit.

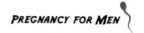

In a very physical sense though, the sixth month marks the beginning of a new chapter when you will be moved gently (at first) away from the mother-to-be of your child. Inch by inch your baby will announce its arrival in your household, your bed and your relationship, by creating its own rotund calling card. The bump is on its way.

There's no getting away from it (and often no getting around it either) – there's an ever-expanding person inside your loved one and it's had the very first announcement from the pilot in the sky to prepare for landing. Before you know where you are, it will be seatbelts on and cross-check to manual.

As the bump arrives, so can three other jolting realisations:

> Pretty soon you are going to have to pay for this person and all its paraphernalia.

> You are going to have to come up with a name for it that neither you nor your partner detests.

> You are going to be a Dad, just like your Dad and his Dad before him.

Bumps, kicks and Braxton Hicks

Does my bump look big in this?

If you are glancing nervously at your partner as you read this thinking, 'She hasn't got much of a bump' for Christ's sake keep that thought in your head and out of your big mouth. The shape, size and position of each bump is as unique as the baby inside it, but that doesn't stop some pretty fierce comparisons taking place between mums-to-be, or even with the odd non-pregger total stranger pitching in to give their tummy two pence as well.

It's also worth forewarning you that the moment your partner begins to show any sign of a bump – that entire area of her body turns into a mobile petting zoo. Old women on buses, old men in trusses, anyone and everyone feels like they can have a little touch. On one level it's quite endearing of course, a very real sign of the shared joy and interest that many of our species still take in the upcoming birth of another of our already numerous clan. It's easy for me to take that philosophical view of course; it's not my stomach being molested.

In terms of advice about the size and shape of the bump though, the only person who is worth listening to about this outward sign of the inward baby is your partner's midwife.

The number of ante-natal check-ups differs from woman to woman, but at each one, the midwife will examine the area by starting under the breastbone and moving down until she feels the top of the womb, an area rather magnificently called the fundus. A measurement is then taken from the top of the pubic bone to the aforementioned fundus and as a rule of thumb, the number of weeks pregnant should roughly correspond to the number of centimetres measured, so at 26 weeks, the bumpage should come in at around 26cm.

If the midwife has any worries whatsoever, she'll get an ultrasound scan jacked up sharpish to check that the baby's growth is normal and put your mind at rest.

The most common factors that could affect bump size are:

> High blood pressure: This causes blood vessels in the placenta to tighten and cuts down on the oxygen that the baby receives. This unsurprisingly sends the little mite into red alert mode and it diverts the available oxygen to its two most important organs – the heart and brain – meaning the rest of the body losses out and can remain small.

> Too much fluid: Too much amniotic fluid could make your bump seem unfeasibly large.

> Not enough fluid: Too little and it appears on the small side.

> Smoking: Smoking reduces the amount of oxygen reaching your baby and women who smoke are three times more likely to have a low birth-weight baby. Smoking in pregnancy is a disaster all round.

> Of course, what's really key to the size of the bump is the size of the baby and the shape of the mummy.

Getting its kicks

It's around now that mothers begin to feel the first fluttering of movement from the baby. Called 'quickening', and described as feeling like the flapping of butterfly wings by those who presumably have spent some quality time with a Red Admiral on their arm, these start to become more noticeable.

From the sixth month onwards for instance, many women start to feel the baby hiccupping as it necks pint after pint of its favourite amniotic brew. As the weeks roll on the frequency and type of movements increase dramatically, as does the basic brute force with which they are delivered.

In the later weeks of pregnancy many a man has been awoken from his slumber by a boot or a jab from within the womb. Waking up startled to realise that your unborn child has just landed one on you is one of life's more surreal experiences. In fact, if ever there's a moment when you realise this tiny thing means business, and will undoubtedly rule your entire life in a matter of months, it's when you also come to on the floor, having been kicked clean out of bed by the little bugger.

In the final few weeks the baby assumes the position, hopefully head down, limiting himself to the odd punch and kick to the ribs as he waits upside down for disembarkation.

Wondering if your baby is kicking enough can cause a fair bit of angst, especially for your partner who is tuned into the baby channel 24 hours a day. The truth is that there are times when the baby wants to rest and times when he wants to play. Studies show that every baby has his own individual pattern of waking and sleeping in the womb. You'll undoubtedly be told by someone that if the baby sleeps during the day and is awake at night you're in for a tough time when he's born, as he will follow the same pattern.

Not only is there no specific scientific evidence to back up that theory, you are also 100% guaranteed to be in a sleepless living hell for at least the first few weeks of parenthood whatever happens, so don't bother worrying about it at this stage and just go to bed while you still can.

This is your father speaking

There was a time, not all that long ago, when leaning into your partner's tummy and talking to your unborn baby was seen as being right up there on the pottiness scale with Prince Charles debating with his dahlias. Now though, scientists are pretty convinced that at around this stage of the pregnancy the baby is capable of learning to recognise the voice of not only his mother-to-be, but his father-to-be too, as well as pieces of oft-repeated music.

A BBC project [16] found that playing the same tune every day for the last trimester of the pregnancy resulted in the baby still recognising (and no doubt being thoroughly sick of it) on hearing it again a year later. Even more astonishing was that an opera singer who took part in the research recounted that she was performing *Aida* while five months pregnant, meaning her unborn son would have heard it non-stop. When, five years later, she was in a production of *Aida* again, her son came to watch her and sat mesmerised through the entire three-hour performance. A five-year-old sitting for three hours at an opera, or indeed anywhere else on the planet, is a feat so unlikely that you can only draw the conclusion, as indeed she did, that somehow he had remembered the music.

So get chatting to your child right now, it's never too early to start the indoctrination process toward your football club – tragically, it can only be a matter of time though before uterine French lessons spring up, with a vocab test taking place five minutes after delivery.

Braxton Hicks – the contraction comedian

You'd imagine the last thing a women needs as she approaches the great unknown of labour for the very first time is her body sending her a few pretend contractions just to keep her on her toes. But that's pretty much what happens in the shape of Braxton Hicks contractions, named after John Braxton Hicks, an English doctor who first discovered this most cruel of all practical jokes in the late 19th century.

Towards the middle of the pregnancy, or sometimes even earlier, your partner may well start to notice the muscles of her uterus tightening for up to a minute or two. Usually painless, they can cause the abdomen to become hard and even contorted, and as the delivery date draws closer they helpfully become more frequent, more intense and more like real contractions, just to really get your partner going. Some women don't get them at all; some poor souls can have them come on several times an hour.

As for why they happen in the first place and what purpose they serve, opinion is divided. Some experts describe them as being a training exercise, a kind of boot camp for the womb, getting it ready for the big push ahead and helping to 'ripen' the cervix so it can go on proper manoeuvres when it's required to. Others though struggle to see how these false contractions, as they are sometimes called, achieve much real physiological value at all. So maybe they are just a bit of a joke?

What isn't very funny is the response your partner will get from midwives and mothers alike if she asks how you can tell the difference between Braxton Hicks and the real deal. Queue rolling eyes, knowing smile and the dramatic, snorting delivery of 'You'll know the difference, don't you worry about that'. How helpful.

What's annoying is that it's true. Labour contractions last longer, are more regular and increase in frequency, as well of course as hurting like the devil himself. A good barometer is that if your partner hasn't told you to rot in hell and never, ever, come anywhere near her again, it's probably a Braxton Hicks she's having.

Of course if you are worried that it might be something more, or the tightness is accompanied by any kind of discharge or lower back pain, get on the blower to your midwife or doctor pronto.

....

Words from your fellow man:

Donald, 34, father of two: *I got on quite well with the bump, spoke to it, played music to it, touched it. But I wasn't very big on touching what was apparently an arm or a leg as it felt a bit awkward for the baby to me, a bit intrusive. My wife on the other hand was much more confident with poking body parts... but it was in her body after all.*

Stuart, 37, father of two: *The bump made me feel a bit scared to be honest, made the whole thing seem a lot more real and nearby. I talked to it a lot and rubbed the stretch mark cream in quite a bit so I wasn't disengaged from it – I was just very aware of what it meant!*

Levi, 36, father of two: *I stroked the bump but felt a proper berk talking to it. I had no such problems the second time around of course, as fatherhood robs you of your dignity anyway.*

Money and lots of it

Are your sitting down? Good. Here are a few financial hometruths for you.

According to various pieces of research, parents in Britain spend an average of £13,696 in their baby's first year, once childcare and loss of earnings are taken into account. Even with many Mums going back to work after 12 months or so, the average baby spend for the second year weighs in at £4,305, and £4,998 for the third year. In fact the average cost of raising a child from birth to the age of 21 has been calculated to be £186,032. That's £738 a month. Every month. For 21 years.

Dry those tears though; it's not all bad news. Once you have children you become eligible for child benefit – £20 a week for your eldest and £13.20 a week for each of your subsequent other children. Woo hoo.

So, it's not cheap then, this parenting carry on. In fact if you were to stare at those figures for too long you'd probably get under the bed and pray to the Almighty that your little one isn't so much born with a silver spoon in its mouth as a diamond-encrusted shovel.

There are of course many ways of keeping costs to a minimum, without resorting to having your baby sleep in a drawer or train as a chimney sweep. Forgive me, but I've presumed that you aren't the type to take a pair of fabric scissors to an old sheet and snip it down to a perfect cot size, or make a crib out of papier mâché and old lentil packets? Thought not; so here's some of the most useful and least time-consuming ways to avoid baby bankruptcy.

The big bad buggy

You may be the kind of man whose right index finger has actually taken on the shape of an Allen key. You may be the kind of man who hides the Screwfix catalogue inside a copy of *Shaven Asian Babes* as you leave the newsagent to avoid any embarrassment. You may even be the kind of man who not only knows which drawer the key to bleed the radiators is in, but also how and when to use it with optimum efficiency.

I'm not that kind of man at all and I'll go as far as to say that far from being an unfortunate and unusual specimen, there are many hundreds of thousands of men like me across Britain. For some reason the line of knowledge about how to put a new blade on the lawnmower, rather than throwing the whole thing away (into the correct skip at the recycling plant of course) has met with a fatal road block at our generation. Were we not listening, or could our fathers just not be bothered to tell us? Who knows? What's for sure though is that for many of us, phrases such as tongue and groove conjure up images of soft porn, rather than DIY.

Of course for most of us this doesn't impact on our lives in any great way, we go about our daily business without the need to read an instruction manual, or construct anything more complex than a club sandwich. Then, just as you are beginning to tackle the not insubstantial issue of your impending fatherhood, the baby buggy looms into view.

I don't want to scare you, I really don't, but this is a world the like of which you will have hitherto never seen. To give you a glimpse behind the wipe-clean curtain of doom, here is a list of just some of the choices that await you when you begin the quest to buy what used to be simply called a pram:

> Three-in-one pram and pushchair combination

> Two-in-one pram and pushchair combination

> Pushchair

> Traditional-style perambulator

> Three-wheeler pushchair

> Travel system

> Pramette pushchair

> All-terrain system

> Buggy

> Stroller

> Tandem

> Double buggy

I could have included the wonderful worlds of car seats and carrycots into the list above but the risk of giving you a brain haemorrhage with the different weight factors, attachment systems and basing units, would be too much for me to cope with, especially with you just about to become a Dad and all.

Once you enter this stroller solar system, there really is no extracting yourself from it – of course you can try to run or avoid it for a while. The technique I desperately clutched at was to collect a few choice baby kit facts and anecdotes and deploy them expertly in the hope of deflecting attention away from the subject. My most successful weapon of mass distraction was: 'The man who came up with the lightweight baby buggy – a Mr Owen Finlay Maclaren – was inspired by one of his previous inventions, the under-carriage for the Spitfire.'

If that failed to derail the conversation I'd unfurl: 'The woman credited with making the Tommee Tippee baby accessory empire the success it is today, was sentenced to eight years in prison in 2007 for plotting to kill her former partner and his wife.'

Not bad are they, and true as well. But in all honesty they only really put off the inevitable for a short while and at some point soon you are going to have to go there too.

If you're waiting for me to tell you which one of these child chariots is best, you are out of luck I'm afraid. Were I to point the finger and even gently criticise any one of the main players, my little boy would be left fatherless within hours as the axis of pushchair evil unleashed its fold-away wrath on me for daring to cast aspersions on one of its members.

What I am prepared to say is this:

> Ask your friends who have already been there and get their advice.

> Newborn babies need to lie back straight, as their malleable spines can be damaged if they are kept curved for any great length of time, so take that into account.

> Think about where your baby is going to sleep as this may affect what you buy.

> If you live in a flat, have a normal sized car, get the bus or train every now and then, or don't happen to have biceps the size of Anglesey, then seriously, seriously think about the size and weight of what you buy. Your back is going to be well and truly fucked as it is carrying a baby around for six months without having to fold and unfold an armoured personnel carrier five times a day too.

What all of these little pointers amount to is a round about way of saying that despite the tedium, the overblown marketing and the colour schemes from hell, it really is worth getting involved in this purchase because with some of the bells and whistles versions getting on towards a £1,000 a pop, this is the single biggest buy you'll make. The number of couples who go through two or even three different versions within the first year alone would make you weep and your bank manager swing for you, if we didn't now own 80% of the company that employed him that is.

The essentials

Where babies are concerned there are a few items, and only a few, other than the dreaded pushchair, that you'll find in every single house that has just taken delivery of a new delivery.

The bed
If you're not careful you can start off with a Moses basket, move on to a carrycot and end up with a fully blown cot before then realising you need a cot bed for your ever-expanding youngster.

Moses baskets are lovely but only useful for a month or two. If you can borrow one, great. Buying a cot that will transform into a small bed is also a smart move. It might seem a long way off, but before you know where you are your defenceless little baby will be vaulting out of his caged pen like a Russian gymnast.

The bath

To a newborn baby being lowered into an adult-sized bathtub is akin to us plucking our eyebrows with a hedge trimmer. Baby baths are worth buying, but remember, it's a plastic bowl that's used to hold water, so the varieties that describe themselves as the ultimate in bathtime pleasure and relaxation for your most precious creation, are probably trying to justify the 30 quid they have lumped onto the price.

The changing mat

Stops your house getting covered in shite – £10 well spent in anyone's book.

Nappies

You'll spend some serious cash on nappies in the first two years. Although there are more and more worried noises being made about the environmental impact of disposable nappies – it's estimated eight million are thrown away in the UK every single day – the chances are it'll be the Pampers and the Huggies you go for, if not initially, then certainly when you begin to realise just how little time for washing re-usable ones you've actually got.

Muslins

This is an absorbent square of cloth usually worn over the shoulder as a badge of honour and used to wipe up all sorts of sticky messes. It has been scientifically proven for it to be impossible to have too many of these in the house – you can have bought three quarters of a million and have every one of them stashed around your two-bedroom flat and it is a cast iron certainty that at the precise moment when you so desperately need one to scoop up a gobbit of milky sick, they will all gather together under the sofa and laugh at you.

Clothes

Babies grow. Babies *really* grow. In the time it takes for you to bend down to pick up one of those disappearing muslins, your child can have grown out of an entire wardrobe full of vests and little socks. It's that fast.

In the first six months if anyone asks what you need, say baby clothes, practical usable baby clothes. It might be dull but for every cuddly crocodile you get given as a gift, you'll wish they'd have spent the spondooliks on two short-sleeved babygros and a pair of mittens to stop them scratching themselves to smithereens in the night with their nails – which also get in on the growing act in quite spectacular fashion.

The real thing to remember is that someone you know will have a binliner full of baby clothes in the loft, just take a little moment to think about it and you will hit romper suit gold. The baby clothes merry-go-round is a British institution, make sure you get on it and you'll save yourself a fortune. And if you don't know anyone with a loft-ful, get onto the Freecycle website (www.freecycle.org) where you can see what people in your neighbourhood are giving away for free, to a good home.

The newcomer

While not strictly essential, the following item has become a firm favourite with Dads in a relatively short space of time and deserves a mention in despatches.

Nappy bins are plastic tubs which house a cartridge in the top that contains a roll of scented nappy bags. Stuff the dirty nappy into the hole, turn the handle and the smelly article has been sealed and can be forgotten about until the bin is full. No trips outside in the middle of the night; no reeking kitchen bin and no leaving them on the stairs for a week.

Be warned. Once your baby starts to eat solids like a grownup they also start to poo like a grownup and the nappy bin begins to struggle to contain its ultra-toxic contents. Eventually the poor bin, after months of sterling service, has to be retired from action and a new plan of attack formulated.

Dig in

No matter how much good advice you're given about saving cash ahead of your new baby's arrival, a strange phenomenon grips both you and your partner. Somehow you forget that you live within a short drive of a supermarket or shopping centre, that whatever you could possibly want on top of the essentials is at most an hour away from being spotted, paid for and transported back to the house. You then begin to buy in everything you will need for the child's entire life. It often starts with buying cutlery for a baby who is still months from being born, let alone moving on to fish fingers. Then it's enormous items of clothing that would swamp a teenager, and jigsaws and books that would test Stephen Hawking.

But in a way this urge to hunker down and get in the provisions is all part of the fun, all part of the excitement of what is about to happen. It feels like Christmas, except you're the ones having Jesus.

But it is though, ultimately, a shocking waste of money. Keeping an eye on eBay, the local charity shop, Freecycle and other websites such as MoneySavingExpert.com (www.moneysavingexpert.com; this website has a huge forum thread dedicated to saving parents cash) will pay fantastic dividends. Madeline Thomas' *Babynomics* (White Ladder,

2010), which looks at all aspects of financing a new family is also well worth a read.

The single biggest stride you need to make though in the battle not to leak cash is that whatever approach you and your partner take, you do your damndest to take it together. There will be enough stresses and strains when the baby arrives without you and your partner falling out about whether Pooh or Tigger should be on the back of the bloody hairbrush you'll never use.

....

Words from your fellow man:

Suki, 34 father of two: *The best piece of kit we bought was the travel system, if you can get one with the carrier that goes straight from the car into the pushchair without waking the baby you will begin to love it like a brother. On the downside the breast pump didn't work very well – but that's obviously second-hand information. Honest.*

Nick, 35, father of two: *We employed a one-stop-shop strategy in terms of getting all the baby stuff. We wrote a long list compiled from talking to a lot of people who'd been there and then went to a baby warehouse where they have everything under one roof. Done and dusted in one go – expect for the things that we forgot – which was almost everything. The one piece of advice I'd give a soon-to-be Dad is never attempt anything without a muslin. It takes me all my might not to take one to work with me nowadays.*

Enzo, 36, father of one: *I found the whole buying for baby thing pretty stressful and very expensive. The marketing people at baby shops are extremely clever. They know parents – particularly the ones who would rather cut both their arms off than scrimp on stuff for their kids – so they screw you for every penny.*

Our very first trip to Mothercare cost us £900 and we only went for a catalogue.

Peter, 33, father of one: *The process of buying all the baby paraphernalia highlights the male/female divide in all its glory. My wife wanted to buy everything and all of it the most expensive. I wanted to try and get bargains. Bottom line in all these arguments was 'she who bears wins'.*

Know your rights – it won't take long

As well as spending money, you'll be wanting to earn a little bit too while you help your new family get to know each other.

If you've not done so already, check to see if your employer has their own paternity leave scheme. If not, you are entitled, if that's the right word, to statutory paternity pay which doesn't make particularly good reading, or indeed spending. You can take up to a maximum of two weeks off and you'll be paid for each of those weeks at £123.06 or 90% of your average weekly earnings, whichever is lower. That's if you meet all the requirements of course; here's one taken straight from a government information website:

'You must have been with your employer for at least 26 weeks by the end of the 15th week before the start of the week when the baby's due.'

All clear? Good.

Things are a bit brighter for your partner though. Many firms have maternity programmes that are better than the statutory agreements, but even the standard terms aren't anywhere near as miserly as what the state offers Dads.

A pregnant employee, under the current statutory guidelines, is entitled to 26 weeks' Ordinary Maternity Leave, followed by a further 26 weeks' Additional Maternity Leave – which adds up to one year in total. As long as the correct notice is given to the employer – more of which below – your partner can take this regardless of how long she's been working there, how many hours she works or how much she happens to be paid.

Statutory Maternity Pay is paid for a continuous period of up to 39 weeks, the first six weeks of which your partner will be paid 90% of her average weekly earnings with no upper limit. For the remaining 33 weeks she will be paid a standard rate of £123.06 per week or 90% of her average weekly earnings, whichever is lower.

You partner is under no obligation to let her employer know she is pregnant until the 15th week prior to the week the baby is due – this is called notification week in the trade and is a time of much rejoicing across the land.

Share and share alike

Some all-round good news on the horizon is that soon mothers who decide to return to work after six months will be able to transfer their remaining six months to the father of the child. As things stand the father would only be paid for three of those six months, but it's certainly a move in the right direction and the plan is for this measure to apply to children due on or after 3 April 2011.

The name game

There are three questions you'll get asked in the immediate aftermath of your child being born and they almost always come in the same order.

1. Boy or girl?
2. What did it weigh?
3. What are you going to call it?

The first two require little thought; a tale and a scale will tell you all you need to know.

What to name your baby though, now there is a real belter of a question and there's a pretty good chance it will have been one that you started arguing over at around this time of the pregnancy. It used to be pretty simple of course, you had a bank of boring but solid names to choose from and choose from them you did. For instance, the top five British boys' names in 1940 were:

1. James
2. Robert
3. John
4. William
5. Richard

In 1950 the list was:

1. James
2. Robert
3. John
4. Michael
5. David

Not what you'd call seismic change over the course of a decade. Of course the war had just ended and people had better things to do than wonder whether 'powdered egg' would sound good as the name of their third daughter.

Of course in many ways now we have gone full circle through the Kylies and the Ethans, and a time when celebrities seemingly arrived at their children's names by picking up the first inanimate object they saw and tarting it up a bit – Plunger Moonlove, Remote Control Angeltears – to a place where the name Jack has been the country's most popular boy's name for a quite frightening 15 years on the bounce, and more girls were called Olivia in 2008 than anything else.

These days, what most of us are searching for when we name our offspring, is something that doesn't have 15 people in the class shouting 'Yes Miss!', when it's called out at registration, but also won't prove be a source of lifelong shame and embarrassment for its incumbent. Tricky.

But does it really matter? Do names really make much of a difference to the life your little one will lead? There's a fair bit of research that suggest the answer could well be yes.

Firstly, a group of 80 experienced teachers were each given four essays, all of similar quality, and asked to mark them. The only identification on them was a first name and a false last initial. The names used were David, Elmer, Hubert and Michael [17]. Before starting their experiment the researchers predicted that the essays 'written' by the children with common, popular names would be graded higher – and their prediction proved to be spot on. The Davids were given the highest marks; the papers by Michael the second highest; those by Elmer the third highest; and poor old Hubert was given the dunce's hat and made to stand in the corner. Poor Hubert.

This study was quickly followed up by another experiment [18] which asked a group of teachers to rate boys' names as desirable or undesirable. The academic achievement scores for the group with desirable names were then compared with the group with undesirable names, and guess what? The average score for the James' was almost twice as high as that of the Arbuthnots – all of which suggests a merry-go-round of inherent and subconscious name-related bias from the teachers and debilitating self-consciousness from the unusually named students.

To put a tin lid on it, recent British research [19] seems to show pretty conclusively that what a child is called really is quite important, with teachers again cast as the name Nazis. This study found that teachers identify troublemakers before they even so much as step foot in the classroom, just by looking down the register. Jacks were considered potential problems, which given the amount of them out there doesn't bode well for the nation's educational well-being, as were boys called Callum and Connor. Alexander and Adam on the other hand were seen as names more likely to belong to the swots. As for the girls, pupils called Chelsea, Courtney and Chardonnay were seen as a potential handful by teachers, but they expected Elizabeth, Charlotte and Emma to be their brightest young ladies.

There are of course a whole raft of names from an ethnic or cultural heritage which are becoming part of the mainstream too, as well as an interesting phenomenon which first started to show itself at the back end of the 90s. For the first time only 50% of babies born in the UK had their names represented in the Top 50 names of recorded births, which means that the other half all had such unique and diverse names that they did not make the charts.

A possible explanation for this is that children born since the mid 1980s are now themselves having children – and if you were given a weird name, why shouldn't your children suffer too?

Lovely.

Snobbery or social science? Whatever's behind it, there's at least a decent case for names having a lifelong impact on us all – so choose carefully wise one, but definitely give Hubert a miss.

Words from your fellow man:

Enzo, 36, father of one: *We both agreed from the outset that we wanted a name that worked both in English and Italian, that being where both of my parents were born. Luckily my wife did not want him named after her father – there is no equivalent of Ken in Italian.*

Levi, 36, father of two: *We had agreed on a shortlist for boys and girls. When the baby was born, I kind of gazumped my wife a bit by telling everyone we'd had a girl and that we thought her name was Rebecca. My wife wanted a good look at her to make sure she suited her name, but by then I'd told everyone anyway. I was right, as it happens.*

Chris, 34, father of one: *We hadn't chosen as we couldn't agree, me liking all those left of field, I-agree-with-Madonna/Gwyneth-*

and-isn't-apple-zuton-mega-faust-sunray-a-great-name, my wife firm on the idea of something that they wouldn't get picked on at school for. We eventually went with Anouk Jasmine – so I won hands down.

Being Dad

Impending fatherhood does many things to a man. It can make him proud of his own virility, see him feel threatened by the new arrival in his kingdom, or render him incontinent with worry about how in the name of Christ he is going to afford it all. There is one aspect of a man's pre-baby processing though that tends to get very little airtime, almost certainly because it involves us talking about how we feel and looking into our past.

As we all know, even now, when the media perception is of millions of new men frolicking around the place trying desperately to embrace their feminine side (as well as anyone who so much as smiles at them), most of us still find the introspection and emotional honesty needed to analyse what really makes us tick a very big ask indeed.

You see, there's nothing like looming paternity to bring back memories of what it was like to be fathered as a child yourself – from snapshots of playing outside, in what seem now like unfeasibly long and sunny summers, to car journeys that whizzed by at the start of the holiday, but made a young and flighty mind almost melt with boredom on the way home. There's a good chance you'll find yourself inexplicably conjuring up all sorts of images as your conscious and subconscious tries to get a handle on the fact that you're next up in Daddy bear's chair.

Of course very few of us grow up guzzling lashings of lemonade in an Enid Blyton world. For many, memories of their father's role in childhood are far from positive. Dread, loneliness, longing, even pain, can be the predominant feelings that this sudden focus on what being a Dad really means can dredge up. For those who experienced a childhood without a father, or lived through male figures coming and going in their life, the prospect of being cast in that role themselves can cause real anxiety and self-doubt. Will they be able to break the pattern, or will what they have always resented about their fathers be the blueprint for how they will raise their own child?

That notion – that as men we are pre-programmed to bring up our children in the same way as our fathers interacted with us, that nature and nurture have already combined to set out our parenting stall for us – obviously has a modicum of genetic truth to it. The clichés about you coming out with a lot of the hackneyed lines your parents fired at you for instance can become horribly accurate all too soon. I'd already said, 'Don't make me come over there' to my son before he had reached his second birthday, which is a shameful thing to have to commit to paper.

The big truth though, according to research, is that no matter how difficult it may be, examining your own childhood and your relationship with your parents means that you are not only much more likely to create your own personal parenting style rather than merely aping the way you were treated, but crucially that you are also much more likely to produce happier and more emotionally adjusted children. Dr Howard Steele of University College London [20] interviewed 100 fathers, whose partners were expecting the couple's first child, to discover how they viewed their own relationship with their parents as they were growing up. Over the course of the next decade many of the men's children were then interviewed and psychologically assessed at various stages of their early life. What became strongly evident was that the initial interviews with the fathers-to-be were powerful predictors of the children's emotional and mental state.

It wasn't though, as you might imagine, a straightforward case of those Dads who had a dire relationship with their own father seeing their children suffer the same fate too. What the study found was that the children whose expectant fathers had really *thought* about the way their parents had related to them were happier. Those whose fathers had responded to the original interview question with ambivalence, or stated that they hadn't really thought about their own childhood in relation to how they were going to approach fatherhood themselves, ended up with offspring who had more difficultly with relationships of all kinds and were generally less happy and more anxious. What also became clear was that although the amount of thought the fathers put into their own childhoods did indeed have a direct link to their own children's mental health, this didn't become apparent until the children hit puberty. Until that point the children's relationships with their mothers seem far more influential. Or to put it in another way, as men we have to put in some serious, considered effort early on, with absolutely no sign of it having any effect whatsoever – and that kind of blind faith, let's face it, is not one of our gender's strong points is it?

That aside, it seems that it's not a case of whether your Dad preferred to stuff you 7–0 at footy in the garden rather than actually play with you; it's more a question of whether you have spent the time reflecting on what a twat he could be at times – or as Dr Steele himself put it in a rather more scholarly way, 'fathers should be encouraged to reflect on their own childhood while their child is still in the womb'.

So if you find yourself drifting back to your early years over the coming weeks, let yourself go, chances are your own kids will thank you for it.

....

Words from your fellow man:

Tom, 34, father of two: *Expecting your own child definitely made me consider the way I was fathered. I remembered all the good times, but I also hoped to be far better in other areas. If the first few years have taught me anything, it's that its bloody hard trying to live up to everything you'd want to be as a father. I just hope I'm not as annoying when I'm 66.*

Peter, 33, father of one: *I definitely made an extra effort with my Dad while we were expecting, but it also highlighted the fact we are not that close – something I don't want to happen with my children.*

Donald, 34, father of two: *You definitely find yourself examining parenthood present and childhood past as the months roll on. You tend to draw similarities and perhaps have a better understanding of what your folks have been through. Did they really deal with all this... was it the same for them... were they more natural... were we just easier kids... (probably not)... or have they just forgotten? You even start dredging up some old sayings from your Mum or Dad, which is scary to hear yourself come out with.*

Enzo, 36, father of one: *When I think of my father I try to picture how happy it would have made him to spend time with his grandson. The fact that Max won't experience that will leave a gap in his life, sadly.*

Levi, 36, father of two: *My Dad died two years before I became a father for the first time and it made me miss him more without a doubt.*

Oli, 35, father of one: *I've never had a Dad around and the constant worry was if we had a boy, would I be good enough, would I know what to do, because I had absolutely nothing to base it on. The worry was less if we had a girl, but still there.*

Move along please

There's another much more intrinsically self-interested and not overly cheery thought which can pop into your head once or twice as you near becoming a father for the first time. You are going to die.

I told you it wasn't cheery. But when you think about it, getting a sense of your own mortality at the point when you are just about to introduce a new life to the planet, isn't all that surprising.

For starters, on a very practical level all of a sudden your death would have a serious impact on the survival of other people – hence your thoughts can turn to wills and life insurance for potentially the first time ever. You might even find yourself driving a bit more carefully, although that's highly unlikely. Then there's the dawning realisation that the start of your son or daughter's childhood will mark the end of your own, in a very real, very, 'I'm too knackered to even think about going out and besides where would we get a babysitter from at this short notice and double besides we can't afford it anyway' kind of a way. While it's not quite one in one out, your offspring's arrival does nudge you along a place towards the end of this earthly plank – or at least it can seem like that in the more contemplative moments that you may well find yourself having as the birth nears.

Don't worry though, nature craftily gives the selfish gene that is the cause of all these 'What about me' thoughts a quick call and flatters the arse off it by first making the baby look like you for the initial few weeks of its life, then a few months later as that little trick is about to wear off, it makes your child not only smile at you, but also start to act like you as well. It's brilliant, and more than makes up for the fact that you are no longer even the second most important person in your own house and have already entered the, albeit gently paced, downhill phase of your very existence.

For now though you are just going to have to trust me as you enter what can be the most inward-looking phase of the pregnancy. Rest assured it doesn't last for long, in a matter of months you won't be giving yourself a second thought as you neglect to shower, shave or eat for three whole days, as you and your partner desperately try to work out why your new baby is screaming like it is being disembowelled with a soup spoon.

Don't be too hard on yourself though, if you can't be introspective on the cusp of the most momentous and important event of your entire life, when can you be? The importance of the role of the Dad in shaping the lives of children has been eroded and underplayed as generations of fathers were forced to spend most of their time at work.

In recent years though study after study [21] has shown that how we perform as fathers profoundly effects how our boys and girls turn into men and women:

> Pre-school children who spend more time playing with their Dads are often more sociable when they enter nursery school.

> Involvement of Dads with children aged 7–11 predicts success in exams at 16.

> Where Dads are involved before the age of 11, children are less likely to have a criminal record by the age of 21.

It's even been found that babies who miss out on regular baths by their father are more likely to grow up with social problems [22]. No pressure then.

The progress report

Month 6 (Baby is 23-26 weeks old)

Your baby

Your baby measures about 23cm from crown to rump and weighs almost 2lbs – his body is now growing faster than his head and his proportions are roughly the same as those of a newborn.

Conscious thought is now possible and your baby can learn and remember – although whether he can hold a grudge at this point remains unclear.

Your baby's ears are going from strength to strength too and he can move his body in rhythm with his mother's voice – like one of those dancing flowers that were all the rage one Christmas a decade or so ago.

It's said that a baby whose father talks to him while he's in the womb can pick out his voice in a roomful of people from birth.

More usefully than mere recognition though, there's a chance he will respond to it too, that is, stop crying when he hears your voice in months to come – now there's an incentive to get talking to that bump if ever there was one.

His nostrils have opened up too, not because he's perfecting a brilliant Kenneth Williams impression to wow you both with on arrival, but because he has begun to make breathing movements with his muscles. He's practising how to breathe.

Won't be long now!

Your partner

The baby's movements and hiccups are now becoming a big part of your partner's existence.

As the baby grows and the womb expands the whole package begins to press on her stomach, exacerbating bouts of heartburn and indigestion as well as rib pain. As her muscles start to stretch and lengthen she may well also get a sharp stitch-like pain down the side of her stomach.

If stretch marks are going to appear, they will make themselves known around now, usually on your partner's stomach or breasts. See this month's must-dos for some advice on handling what, as you can imagine, is a very delicate topic.

Now is also the time that pelvic floor muscles start to become stretched. The oft talked about pelvic floor helps to hold your partner's bladder, womb and bowel in place – so it's worth having. The muscles also act as the valve mechanism that allows her to empty her bladder and bowels. Trouble is being pregnant can make these muscles become very weak or overstretched and can result in a little bit of wee leaking out when she coughs, exercises or laughs. Tips on how to help her strengthen these muscles follow shortly, but for now just remember that every gag you tell her from this point onwards has the potential to be literally piss funny.

THE MUST-DOS OF THE MONTH

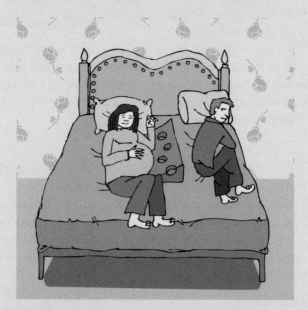

Give her a wedgie

Stick 'pregnancy wedge pillow' into Google, and if she hasn't already got one, buy one. She gets to support her bump in bed, and yet again you look like the best father-to-be a gal could ever wish for.

At a stretch

Stretch marks affect between 75% and 90% of pregnant women. The combination of more weight and higher levels of hormones making the skin thinner than usual is a pain, and can cause some serious anguish and anxiety for many women both during and after pregnancy.

Tips to help keep the skin healthy and supple abound: rubbing the skin with olive oil, vitamin E-rich cream or royal jelly, and drinking lots of water.

There's a good chance though that despite your loving and magic fingers your partner may well develop a permanent stretch mark or two. Your role then is simple; tell her you love her and that she is beautiful, every single day.

Floor it
In motivational terms, the reasons for your partner doing pelvic floor exercises are about as compelling as they come. These exercises help:

> Protect her from incontinence during and after the pregnancy

> Support the extra weight of pregnancy and may even help shorten the second stage of labour

> Heal the perineum after birth

> Achieve orgasm during sex.

Makes you wonder why we aren't all doing them en masse in the work car park every morning.

Like most things that are good for you these exercises are far from a doddle to do though. Most advice seems to centre around your partner imagining she is stopping herself from passing wind and weeing at the same time – so as a man this is way out of your comfort zone lavatorially speaking.

If you are still enjoying some mid to late pregnancy nookie then you can be of even more help. If your partner does the lift and squeeze movement while you are inside her, your penis can act as a detector rod and you can cheerfully inform her if you can feel her efforts.

Romance? Dead? Get outta here.

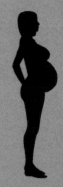

MONTH 7
Brace yourselves

You are well and truly in the third trimester, which means the final preparations are about to begin and you are going back to school.

That's right: it's time for you to experience the antenatal class in all its glory: the breathing exercises, the vaginal discharge conversations, the pressure to meet lifelong friends in a handful of hours. I'm excited for you, I really am.

Then there's a very different form of preparation to tackle, trying to get your head round how having a baby will change your relationship.

In many ways it's one of the most important yet neglected areas of the pre-birth period. We all focus heavily on the moment of the birth and how to deal with the baby that pops out as a result of it, but often people don't give a second thought to how this new little being will change the bond they have with the person they made it with.

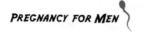
The antenatal experience

Rite of passage or right pain in the arse?

Antenatal classes often draw differing and extreme responses from fathers-to-be. Some can't imagine attempting to tackle the trials and technicalities of birth without the crash course they receive while sitting cross-legged on the floor of a local church hall. Others would do anything to get out of them, praying that extreme weather will force the primary school-style cancellation of their torment.

Although there are many types of antenatal class around these days they tend to come in two distinct flavours: the antiseptic hand gel NHS version and the pumpkin soup with a hint of saffron private variety of which the National Childbirth Trust (NCT) classes are by far the most predominant.

Typical classes, whether NHS or NCT, often follow a course over six to eight weeks, with the majority of women in attendance due to give birth at roughly the same time.

NHS antenatal classes

It's usual, but by no means certain that if you choose to go down the NHS route you'll have your classes at the hospital you are booked in to deliver the baby. These are usually free of charge and taught by midwives who not only tell you about every detail of labour and birth but also about that particular hospital's policies and procedures.

Information will include what labour is like, what pain relief can and can't do, sessions on the prospect of interventions, explanation of the clinical name for when someone comes at your wife wielding a pair of forceps or a plunger-like device (a Ventouse, of which there is much, much more in Month 9) and caesarean (c-section) births. You might also be taught a few parenting skills, for example how to bath a baby and change a nappy and crucially where you'll find CBeebies on Freeview, Freesat and Sky.

They may also give you the opportunity to have a tour of the maternity unit, which is worth doing for sure, but is a bit like being given a detailed look at your dentist's tray of shiny instruments before he sorts out your root canal. NHS classes are often large and a bit more impersonal than their privately organised cousins, but then this is the NHS, God bless her, so a comfy chair, coconut macaroon and foot massage were never really on the cards were they?

Just to give you a taste of things to come, you may not be taught by the same midwife for each class, as their day (and night) job can be a tad unpredictable, meaning they have to hand over to whoever is free.

NCT antenatal classes

NCT classes are the undisputed king of private antenatal tuition. Other organisations hold them and plenty of former midwives have set up their own sessions too, but with more than 1,000 qualified teachers and an army of 10,000 volunteers, the NCT is the alpha female of the antenatal world.

Founded in 1956, the NCT looked to challenge the childbirth orthodoxy of the time, which was essentially that women kept quiet and did what their (almost certainly male) doctor told them. One of the organisation's original published aims gives us a pretty good indication of what having a baby was like back then: 'Women should be humanely treated during pregnancy and in labour, never hurried, bullied or ridiculed.'

Ridiculed! Bloody hell, what did these doctors do, stand around the bed shouting ' 'ark at her at her, moaning and screaming, boo, hoo, hoo'?

Another founding principle states that analgesia should not be forced on women in childbirth – or, please stop rendering women unconscious with chloroform the first time they so much as ask for a glass of water.

With these kind of values at its beating heart, it's no surprise that the NCT has evolved into the champion of natural childbirth and for that matter breastfeeding over bottle – and is unashamedly women-centred. Equally unsurprising is the fact that its antenatal classes reflect that ethos, which has led to them gaining a knit-your-own-lentils, earth-mothery reputation from some quarters. How accurate that reputation is, is highly debatable and it seems everyone in the pregnancy realm has a take on it.

What is for certain is that the NCT antenatal classes remain incredibly popular. Instructors are not usually midwives, but women who have had at least one baby. They aren't just grabbed off the streets though you'll be glad to hear, they have all been trained in what they do and most deliver the classes within an informal setting, which can quite often be their own home. Small class sizes add to the friendly feel as does the often hands-on teaching style, which can see your partner, and often you too, practising relaxation skills and different positions for labour, as well as receiving information on the ins and hopefully outs of the birth itself and all the scenarios that surround it.

Costs start at around £120 per course and can rise to £300 depending on where you live, but being the good eggs they are, the NCT has a raft of payment plans and discounts to try to make it possible for almost everyone to take part in one of its classes if they want to.

With their more intimate air and informal approach, NCT classes and their ilk have taken on an interesting subtext in recent years too, one far away from the mere imparting of knowledge and information. As you arrive at your first class, looking round the room at the glowing women and sweaty just-come-from-work men, there's a fair chance you'll think two things. Firstly, I hope I don't have to take my shoes off because I think my left sock has a hole in the big toe, and, secondly, at least two couples in this room need to become our new best friends. It's the unspoken law of the antenatal class that because the two main stars of modern adult friendship are aligned, namely:

> Do we have something, anything, in common – err yes, something quite large and round?

> Do we live near each other – probably.

You would somehow have to be a complete social nightmare not to bond and develop a long-lasting connection with at least some of the people at these classes.

And don't forget, this isn't just friendship for friendship's sake, this is about developing a support network, no, a vital support network for your partner as she struggles alone at home after you've gone back to work.

So don't balls it up alright. Oh dear.

Your journey begins with the chit-chat before the start of the first class. Despite your best laid plans you and your partner find yourself sitting next to the strange pair who bring their own sandwiches and sport facial hair (yes both of them), while the three cool but not showy couples stand in a little huddle talking and laughing. Oh how they laugh.

The preamble ends and the couples sit facing each other. You are now utterly desperate to make amends for your poor positional play at the start of the proceedings. You decide to make an impression using your famous sense of humour, but realise too late that a tortuous tale about how much you find your partner and indeed pregnant women in general sexy, has made you sound like a dirty dog rather than the sensitive soul you had hoped for.

Now on a damage limitation footing, you keep schtum for the remainder of the class. As things draw to a close you see two of the women swapping numbers and their husbands even mention meeting up for a beer. It's a disaster, as friendships are forged all around you, your partner beckons for the door and you slink out vowing to make a real impression next week and erase your newly acquired reputation as a pregnancy pervert.

It needn't be like this of course, and please God it won't be. You may for instance be the couple with facial hair who operate on a higher plain and aren't crippled with insecurities like the rest of us, or failing that at least have remembered to put on a new pair of socks.

However it plays out, there's no getting away from the fact that antenatal classes now come with an added and unspoken pressure that means not only have you got to massage your partner's feet in public, you've also got to use the same hand to deliver a firm handshake to the other Dads that says, 'Yes, this is a man I want to escape to the pub with in six months time.'

To go or not to go?

There was a time, not so long ago, when men just didn't do things like go to pre-pregnancy classes. There was no point – they certainly weren't going to be at the birth and as for knowing how to change a nappy well, they might as well be shown their way round a set of curling tongs so unlikely was it that they would be called upon to carry out that task. But times have changed and you have to be a real throwback not to attend on purely gender-based grounds now. Even Australian men are being encouraged to go, albeit via a newly formed scheme that has started to hold classes in pubs so as to be 100% sure of attendance [23].

But is it worth the effort for either of you? Do these classes teach you anything of value or are they just a racket, which in the case of the private versions extract cash you can ill afford to spend, just to tell you what you could have learned from a book very much like the rather splendid one you have in your hands at this very moment? The answer for many is yes, of course it's worth the effort.

While we all might occasionally attempt to put up a coffee table with scant regard for the instructions, the thought of going through labour without at least a few pointers about what in the name of jumping Jesus is going on is increasingly too terrifying for many men to comprehend.

Will what you learn make the experience less painful for your partner?

Probably not. (A recent survey found that antenatal classes that put emphasis on breathing and relaxation techniques don't make a blind bit of difference to the number of women who end up needing an epidural or caesarean [24]).

Will the classes mean you play a more useful role in the delivery room, rather than standing around like a complete tool asking if everything is alright when it patently isn't? Nope, that's your job.

Will you learn to see childbirth as a beautiful and spiritual experience that in itself will enrich your life forever? No, because while it's memorable, it's often shocking in equal measure.

But none of that matters. What antenatal classes really do is make you think you are pretty well prepared for what's to come; they make you believe you have a handle on whatever will come your way and even though that is a complete load of bollocks, it's all you've got so cling on to it.

Besides, it's a great place to make new friends, honest.

Words from your fellow man:

Peter, 33, father of one: *I would recommend NCT classes to everyone – best £120 I've ever spent. You pick up a few things but the main thing was my wife picked up seven like-minded women, who in the run-up to the birth and the first year of having the little one have been invaluable. Of course the two of you together are the most important people to make sure you get through, but never underestimate the relief you get from speaking to people facing the same daunting baby mountain as you.*

Tom, 34, father of two: *Antenatal classes are worth doing for so few reasons. Sure we met a couple of nice people, but keeping up with your own bestest friends is hard enough, especially when you are on permanent baby duty. Usual mix at ours I guess,* with a couple of annoying ones for good measure. The one thing I recall is that if a dog licks your baby's face it won't really affect it. Everything else was a battle to stay awake, let alone be interested in. But it was a key milestone, it meant we were in the final run in, and this is the best bit about NCT. It gets you in the zone, and it's nice to have others to share it with.

Jim, 34, father of one: For some reason I got severe indigestion whenever we went to an antenatal class (thank God for the herbal tea). I also always forgot all the names, all of the time, but they were good fun when I was awake. And the teacher was supportive after the birth, bless her.

Nick, 35, father of two: We attended one class – and it was not a good experience. I had to hold an item picked from a bag and explain why it was relevant. I got a plastic pear. It apparently meant that I had to remind my wife to eat lots of roughage after the birth to ensure she was regular. I didn't go again.

Birth choices – who does the best delivery?

If you do decide to take part in antenatal classes of any description they are certain to throw up as many questions as they provide answers, especially when it comes to the type of environment your partner should deliver her baby in.

Home births

In 1955, there were 683,640 births in England and Wales, of which 33.4% took place at home. In 2006, of the 662,915 babies born, a mere 2.7% arrived at home, the vast majority born in hospitals and other medical institutions.

Eminent zoologist Desmond Morris in his brilliant little book *Babywatching* [25] suggests that this shift towards medical institutions constitutes a major difference in the labour human females endure and to the relatively relaxed way in which our close cousins in the animal kingdom deliver their young. Morris proposes that because modern mothers-to-be are rushed off to a strange and daunting place with strong associations with illness and pain and then put in the hands of relative strangers, they become, understandably, anxious.

Just as nine out of 10 pregnant horses give birth in the dead of night – the mare instinctively waiting until the least stressful part of the day – Morris suggests that women subconsciously and hormonally struggle with the same intuition too, which results in labours many times longer than normal for our species.

He goes on to say that while home births are of course possible, so out of the norm have they become that they themselves now carry bucketfuls of anxiety too – with mothers worried that they are too far away from the expert help that hospitals afford.

It's a very interesting theory and one which makes much sense. But the fact remains that while moves have been made to promote home births they still represent a tiny minority, especially of first babies. If you would like to explore a home birth, talk to your midwife if you haven't already.

Birthing units

So the statistics say that you will almost certainly go for, or end up having, a hospital delivery. Luckily there's now some choice in this area too, with the advent of the midwife-led birthing centre. These units often feel cosier, more relaxed and less clinical than a regular hospital and some say they even bridge the gap between giving birth at home and on a hospital maternity ward.

The obvious drawback, if indeed you see it as a drawback, is that with a somewhat low-tech approach centred on birthing pools, balls and stools, comes fewer choices on the pain relief front. For instance your partner will have to be transferred to a hospital if an epidural is needed (although often this is essentially an internal transfer as the birthing centre is attached to the hospital itself).

Going private

Can you buy a better birth? Some people with anything up to 10 grand burning a hole in their pockets seem to think you can.

There's a range of private birth units across the UK, offering private rooms, state-of-the-art facilities, one-to-one care during labour and beyond, top-notch meals and what is marketed as the most peaceful, relaxed and personal way to have a baby. It's worth bearing in mind though that depending on the unit there's a good chance that in the event of a medical emergency your partner would need to be transferred to an NHS hospital.

Costs vary, but when you start to add in the consultant's fees and extra nights after the birth you are talking about many thousands of pounds for the privilege.

A cheaper alternative is to book a private room in an NHS hospital for use after the birth. Often called amenity rooms, these are private rooms situated on or close to the postnatal wards. Midwives tend to allocate them on the basis of clinical need, but it is possible to book one depending on availability. If the birth is uncomplicated your partner may well just be allowed to go back home the next day, but after something like a caesarean section these can represent a viable option. Costs vary widely from hospital to hospital, with some coming in at under £100 a night, and others many hundreds of pounds.

Howdy partner

Another area that your antenatal classes may bring into focus is who will be your partner's birthing partner. If at this point you are shouting at the book, 'Birthing partner? *I'm* the bloody birthing partner!' then you are probably clear that you will indeed fill that role and good on you.

But increasingly there are other options that are coming into the mix. Your partner may want some girl power in the room and her mum, sister or best friend may be who she wants there as well as, or even instead of you. Tough luck. As we will see in Month 9, there's plenty for the birth partner to do, some critical decisions to act as the mother-to-be's advocate on in fact – and it's this scenario that has largely given rise to the paid-for birth partner, or doula.

Doulas almost always have experience in the delivery environment and offer continuous support and guidance throughout labour. They can either be an additional birth partner or the sole companion. It's obviously imperative that you choose one which both your partner and you get on with and can see yourself working well with under one of the most pressurised situations you will ever face.

The number of doulas working across the UK has increased in recent years, with around 1,000 operating currently, but there are still no specific qualifications needed to work as one – anyone can do it. So finding out what experience and training they have before you plump is also vital. Charges vary widely, the going rate being anything from £300 to about £800, depending on the doula's experience. The fee often includes antenatal and postnatal visits as well.

Your relationship – all change please

It's often said that women have an unwritten rule when it comes to telling their thus-far-childless female friends about the reality of labour. They lie.

Whether it's a Darwinian instinct to protect the future of the species by not scaring people away from procreation, a schadenfreudian desire to see someone else go through the same agony as they have, or just good manners, no woman ever tells it like it really is in the delivery room.

There is, however, a male version of this phenomenon, and I'm about to reveal it. There's no easy way of putting this so I'll just come right out and say it: there's a very good chance that your relationship as you know it will very shortly end for good. That's not to say you and your partner won't be together, nor that you won't be happy; it's just that what you've had in the past and are currently enjoying the Indian summer of, will never be the same again. Ever.

For many couples the months and sometimes years after they first become parents usher in a period of such upheaval that it can feel as if at the moment their child arrived the person they thought they knew back to front disappeared and was replaced with someone who looked remarkably similar, but acted very differently indeed. At the heart of this conundrum is one key question: can a truly equal partnership, the kind that most women and indeed men expect in these enlightened times, exist when a baby arrives who hasn't a clue about gender roles and equality movements, but quite likes the look of those breasts?

When studies of British parents find that far from bringing happiness and joy, an increasing number of modern Mums and Dads feel that the arrival of their offspring has left them feeling 'angry and resentful' [26] and even 'miserable, sad, distracted and depressed' [27], it's hard to avoid the conclusion that something is going on here. Then there's the earlier work, undertaken in the USA, which followed more than 300 couples having their first child over a period of six years [28]. The studies, which documented in greater depth than ever before the amazingly stressful social and emotional consequences of parenthood, revealed that for about half of the couples who participated, marital satisfaction declined after the birth of a first child.

Of course, having children has always been a challenge; always upset the apple cart, even in the days when the apple cart was the very height of commercial transportation technology. For your average newborn things are pretty much as they were: babies have always cried; always been a bit lax on the toilet front; always had an idiosyncratic (some might even say downright quirky) sense of day and night; and have always, always, been the centre of attention in their household.

But we – that's you, me and everyone who is having children today – are right in the middle of a seismic shift in the very way the family unit works. The foundations of the partnership men and women enter into when they start a family are moving under our feet, leaving both partners on shaky ground. Before we look into exactly how and why the modern-day relationship all too often suffers a temporary cardiac arrest when children arrive – and crucially how you can avoid it flat-lining altogether – it's worth taking a look at how being a father has evolved into what it is today. Pay attention at the back.

A short history of Dad

Fathers haven't got a great reputation historically. The hands-on Dad or 'new man' phenomenon is widely seen as just that, new; with the father figure of yesteryear almost universally viewed as a pretty uncaring beast.

> Prehistoric Dad: An idyllic existence for the loin-clothed old man, hunting and gathering during the day, sharing a cave with scantily clad wife(s) by night. Little interest taken in Bam-Bam-like infant. Occasional sabre-tooth tiger attacks the only blot on landscape.

> Medieval Dad: Saxon fathers had a tendency to pelt offspring with parsnips when displeased with them. Aside from this occasional vegetable abuse, the father was a peripheral, pox-addled figure.

> Elizabethan Dad: Good practice for a father consisted of throwing their young into a woven sack, transporting them to the docks and selling them to barnacle-covered explorers as tobacco tasters and potato smokers.

> Victorian Dad: Children spent the majority of their time

strapped into metal frames and forced to permanently pose for 10-hour box brownie photo shoots, leaving father plenty of time to cultivate his already impressive opium habit.

> 1950s Dad: Children beaten by fathers for questioning authority figures.

> 1960s Dad: Children beaten by fathers for not questioning authority figures.

> 1990s and the noughties: Dads finally begin to get it and start to take interest in their young. The emergence of man-bags signals that the shift has gone too far, but a crisis is averted.

The reality though is very different. Adrienne Burgess, author of *Fatherhood Reclaimed* (Vermilion, 1998), paints a picture of historical fatherhood that bears very little resemblance to the way most of us imagine it to have been. Our view of the hunter-gatherer in primitive societies spending most of the time slaying wild boar far away from home is a dodgy one for starters. In most tribes fathers were present for the majority of the time and in many there developed a pride among men that they were close to their children.

Jump forward an epoch or two and rural Dad wasn't too shabby on the childcare front either. With life regulated by daylight, fathers were only away from a lighted house or cottage for a handful of hours while in summer the whole family often worked together in the fields. Even in more wealthy families, children often slept in the same room as their parents; the nursery room tucked away in the attic didn't start to appear until much later.

Then there are the stats – after formal/informal divorce, fathers often won custody of their children and when you take into account that around 8% of mothers died in childbirth, many more men than women were lone parents. In fact it's estimated that between

1599 and 1811, 24.1% of children lived in lone father households, compared with just 1.3% today! So what the hell happened to catapult us to the world where waiting until your father got home became something to be feared rather than looked forward to? You guessed it global warming fans: the sooty paw prints of the industrial revolution are all over it.

The main way in which both physical and emotional distance has been put between fathers and their children is through the idea of the father as sole provider for the entire family. The man-as-breadwinner model might seem as old as the family unit itself to us now, but it wasn't until the steam-driven late 19th century that bringing home the corn began to be seen as the male's *raison d'être*.

But rejoice my brother, because fathers are making a comeback. After more than 200 years of being set apart from our own families, cast as the provider but never carer, we're trying our best to become a true part of it all again, which is great, obviously; but far from straightforward. You see, while we've been trying to change, wrestling ourselves away from our desks, diggers and dustcarts, and moving heaven and earth to make it home for bath time, things have changed at home too – in a big way. Being a 'husband' in Britain is in many ways unrecognisable from how it was just 50 years ago for one woman-sized reason – being a 'wife' has been utterly transformed too.

Woman, wife/partner, mother

When I was five years old, my Dad walked into our house one summer's evening and proudly told us all that the family had a new car. By new he meant a very old Austin Princess but that's a minor point – what's interesting now that I look back to that day in the late 1970s is that this revelation was news to my mother too. My father had sold our old car and bought a new one without consulting with my Mum and it didn't so much as raise a matrimonial eyebrow.

Do you know a man under 40 who has done anything even remotely like that? If so please do pass on to them my sense of awe and tell him that arnica is meant to be excellent for bruises.

The car was Dad's domain together with providing for the entire family, filling out the pools coupon and getting the fire going. Bringing up the children on a day-to-day basis, running the house and keeping everyone fed, washed and watered was what Mum did. Thank you and goodnight.

Now please don't imagine for a second that I'm pining for those days again – but by Christ things were a whole lot more straightforward then. You don't need to be a social historian, or indeed a woman, to see that the clearly defined gender roles which many of our parents and all of our grandparents operated within have changed profoundly and forever. It's only a handful of decades, for instance, since the stipulation for a woman being granted a mortgage was that she must get either her husband's or her father's signature. A woman was her father's daughter before becoming her husband's wife.

No longer of course, at least not in many parts of the world. The women's movement turned all the old assumptions about the roles of the genders on their head, a shift which also coincided with a fundamental change in the very nature of work itself. As the old heavy industries were replaced with knowledge-based jobs, the need for brawn and physical strength was replaced with the need for people who were at ease with human interaction and emotion, as well as being able to carry out more than one task at a time. Now let me think, which gender would that suit best?

Professional satisfaction as well as personal and sexual freedom is within the grasp of today's women in a way never seen before and ambitions don't just centre on being wives or mothers. This in turn has also had a subtle effect on the laws of attraction and partner selection. Whether your potential wife is a good cook, keeps the house nice and tidy or has child-bearing hips are questions that have been consigned to the dustbin of male chauvinist history. Now we look for partners not cleaners; it's a soulmate we want, someone who we can share our lives with; a companion.

When we've found that special person, often nowadays someone who earns as much or more than we do, life can feel pretty sweet for both parties. Every couple is different of course, but in the main the number of relationships in which the man could change the family car without by your leave to his partner is falling rapidly. A more typical scene now would be hours of joint internet research, followed by much debate and list drawing before they finally reach a compromise or go with one choice over another, leaving the loser to persistently pick holes in the wretched automobile for the next five years. A palaver for sure. But a relatively fair and equal one.

It's no surprise then that faced with the opportunity to establish a career, achieve some level of financial security, be part of a true partnership with someone and just have a bloody good time, the average age of the first-time mother has jumped to 30 and counting. Foreign holidays, cool careers, good food, – oh yes, this is what dreams are made of, this is what relationships have evolved into, this is what real equality between the genders can bring.

And then you have a baby.

A nappy-wearing cluster bomb lands right in the middle of your serene and blissful partnership, and not having read much Germaine Greer or indeed giving a toss about the hard-fought gains of the feminist crusade, his prime concern is to be fed, winded and changed. Now.

The ideology of equality that many of us now live by within our relationships has come on leaps and bounds for sure – but babies, tiny, innocent little mites with not much on their minds but milk, have the power to shake your new and happy world to the core.

What also makes this such a tricky situation to manage is that, in a very real sense, we are pioneers; the first generation to feel the full effect that a baby, with his needs and habits honed over thousands of years, can have on a modern relationship. Your Dad can't help you, your older brother can't help you, even the bloke at work with three teenage kids doesn't really understand. To a greater or lesser degree they all lived in a straightforward, almost quaint, world that we can only look back on like some strange Inca civilisation.

No, it's down to us to work out how to stop the baby bomb from causing some serious collateral damage in our households, and what follows is some of the fallout to watch out for. Thinking about it ahead of time may not provide you with all the answers, but looking after your first baby is tough enough without being blown away by the sheer shock of how much the rest of your life seems to have changed too.

Turn and face the strange

So, things are going to change, but how?

Here's a whistle-stop tour of the two main areas in which your bundle of joy will indirectly alter how you and your partner get along. If, in the early weeks and months of being a father you spot one of this troublesome pair, and chances are you will, you might just stand a chance of summoning up the time, forethought and energy to adjust what you are about to say or do and avoid a flashpoint that everyone could do without, especially the smallest one of your trio.

It's a sad irony that some conscientious parents these days put in a lot of effort to ensure their new baby has every gadget and gizmo he could possibly need to make him comfortable and happy in his early days, but then proceed to argue and bitch around the little mite for six months as they become engulfed by the huge changes he brings on how they previously worked as a couple.

I blame the conspiracy of silence that has resulted in men and women being led blindly into this brave new world. But no longer...

Bond, maternal bond

Everyone knows that mothers and babies bond. It's one of nature's staples, like needles playing hide and seek in haystacks and bears using woods as their toilet. There's no two ways about it, early on babies only have eyes, ears and nostrils for Mum and often the same is true in reverse.

For many new fathers this can hit home more than they ever imagined it would. Feelings of jealousy towards this unfeasibly cute little intruder who has so besotted their loved one are well chronicled and while for some men this can be a real problem, what is much more common is the feeling of total and utter uselessness that washes over new, keen and achingly well-informed new Dads. You've done the antenatal course, you've watched the DVD, you've even bought a bloody book for crying out loud, but the 50/50 spilt you employed before the arrival of the little one is often nowhere to be seen.

This one-sided scenario, as we will see in a short while, can cause problems aplenty for your partner too, but in the first few weeks it's the Dads who run the risk of feeling like they've put a lot of thought into what to wear to a party, only to be asked to wash up when they get there. That's a pretty stark picture of course and you may not feel as edged out early on – your partner may even have had a caesarean in which case you'll be a very busy boy indeed, but no matter what your personal circumstances are, there's a strong chance that you'll feel a little sidelined as the overwhelmingly powerful surge of love between baby and mother kicks in.

When you stop for a second to compute the fact that just the sight, smell and sound of her baby can make a woman flood the place with the milk she needs to support him, you can see that Mums make decisions at this extraordinary point in their lives based on instinct, an instinct that just days before didn't exist. There are no brochures to consult, no googling the answer, she often just knows, feels, what is right for the baby at this crucial early stage and you as the father just plain don't.

There will be conversations of course, even the odd compromise, but when push comes to shove, your partner will almost always back her intuition to tell her the right thing to do by the new arrival. It's the way it is and always has been. That's not to say all women know what to do from the off, harnessing this intuition, this feeling, can be an overwhelming and daunting task in itself.

When you consider that it was only around 100 years or so ago that infant mortality rates in the fantastically prosperous UK were at levels that would turn even the most relaxed of women into fiercely protective sabre tooth tigresses, it's a wonder we are allowed to stay under the same roof, let alone be tolerated to suggest that it might be good to give the week-old tot his first bath.

In the mid 1950s, eminent paediatrician, psychiatrist and psychoanalyst Donald Winnicott identified and highlighted this early state of intense mother–baby bonding, naming the phenomenon primary maternal preoccupation [29]. Winnicott observed a special mental state of the mother that involved a greatly increased sensitivity to, and focus on, the needs of her baby, starting near the very end of pregnancy and continuing for a few weeks after the birth.

It's also been noted that not only does a mother need support and protection while she is in this phase, but that the benefits of the secure attachment it creates can have positive effects on the child right through childhood and into adult life. Which is a polite way of saying, butt out numb-nuts. But what's key to remember is that the early days and weeks of your new family's existence are like no other. No matter what plans you had made, no matter how interwoven you and your partner were before the arrival, nature is calling the shots; and although you play a very important role in those early days, you are very much the best supporting actor rather than the joint lead.

Fear not though, the time when you will be expected to step up to the plate is just around the corner, bringing with it another set of challenges to negotiate.

Jobs and doing them

After the first few weeks of a baby's arrival things start to get back to normal. Well, not normal, just a different kind of different.

What stops are the visits from friends and relatives and the arrival of presents. Even the nice old woman from over the road comes round to collect the dish she brought the shepherd's pie in during the baby's first week at home.

What starts is the graft. It's hard to overestimate the wonder/panic you'll feel at how such a small and defenceless little thing can generate so much work for two adults. This outrageously increased workload also sits against a backdrop of complete and utter knackeredness.

It's hard to put into words just how exhausted you'll be:

FUUUUUUUUUUUUUUUUUUUUUUUCCCCCCCCCCCCCCCCC KKKKKKKKKKKKKKKKKKKKKKKKKKKKKED was the best I could come up with.

Sleep deprivation has been used as a means of interrogation, most famously by the KGB. Menachem Begin, the Prime Minister of Israel from 1977 to 1983, who was unfortunate enough to have experienced the technique while a prisoner in Russia, described it as follows [30]:'In the head of the interrogated prisoner, a haze begins to form. His spirit is wearied to death, his legs are unsteady, and he has one sole desire: to sleep.... . Anyone who has experienced this desire knows that not even hunger and thirst are comparable with it.'

Yep, that sounds about right.

Then there's the fact that you will almost certainly be back at work too, thanks to the pathetic paternity leave we are all graciously granted. Deep joy.

So, with all those ingredients in the pot we have a potentially explosive situation on our poo-covered hands. Here's how it tends to work.

After a pitiful amount of sleep you make your way to work like a mole with a bad headache. Your equally shattered partner spends the entire day with a life form that is only capable of doing the following things: eating, crapping, vomiting and crying. Not surprisingly pretty soon the charm of this four-pronged approach wears a little thin and your partner, now permanently smelling of regurgitated milk and drowning under a sea of off-white cotton clothing, asks you to help out more – to not only do your fair share but above and beyond that too. Slightly stung you swallow hard and try to do what you think is being asked of you, be more proactive and take some of the pressure off your partner. Now's not the time, you are proud of yourself for thinking, to point out that between the hours of 8am and 6pm you are actually working, rather than as she seems to be implying being massaged for 10 hours while watching the cricket. So you get involved more, which often leads to two things happening.

Scorekeeping

This is a game invented by the devil. To start off with both you and your partner keep a secret tally in your heads of the chores you've performed over the course of let's say a week. On the unspoken scoreboard you are getting murdered of course, absolutely hammered out of sight. In nappy changing alone you are down by more than 40 points and if she's breastfeeding as well, my word, you might as well pack up and go home. Except you can't because that's where the game is being played.

Then one day, after you have yet again put one of the few nappies you have changed *on* the bin rather than *in* it, she explodes and proceeds to douse you in a torrent of pent-up point scoring. You attempt to come back of course: you de-iced the car the other day, and so often are you spotted late at night in the supermarket that the security staff are beginning to become suspicious. But it's a feeble defence, she's at home with the baby and therefore does the lion's share of the baby stuff. Stands to reason doesn't it?

Under no circumstances point that out. None whatsoever.

You see this isn't really about who does what, it's about your partner's expectation and reality of motherhood smashing into each other like they have been sent round the Large Hadron Collider. It's a snapshot of the schism we are in as a generation when it comes to the roles of men and women. After years of progress to gain sexual equality, this tiny throwback lands in the household and not only is the woman forced to put the career she's worked so hard to achieve on hold, she also now finds herself spending her days wondering what would best remove faeces from sheepskin. It's an enormous shift and what compounds it is how things look from the other side of the fence. After doing your best to be useful at the labour you have a fortnight off work to glory in the gifts and the visits that a beautiful new baby attracts before slotting, albeit wearily, back into your old life.

With this kind of hellish dance going on there's little wonder surveys are finding that relationships are struggling to survive with this kind of deep dissatisfaction and resentment knocking about.

As a mechanism for rationalising the new world they find themselves in, many new mums are subconsciously doing something quite ingenious to redress the balance: they formulate the practical side of motherhood into a work-like format, a job – and that, my friend, makes them the boss and you an employee.

The emergence of the manager Mum

Show me a successful company and I'll show you a building full of bright, conscientious hard-working women. There might still be discrepancies on the pay front, but when it comes to capability, only the most arse pinching, cleavage ogling fool of a man would fail to admit that over the past 50 years women really have if not conquered the workplace, then certainly populated and propagated it.

Today's working woman defines herself not by the shine of her front step, or the brilliant whiteness of her net curtains, as many of our mothers and certainly grandmothers may well have done, but by how she performs and how she is perceived to perform in her career. Taking that away and replacing it with Cbeebies is one hell of a physiological smack in the solar plexus. So what do many of these capable and confident women do to compensate? They manage their new job, that of rearing a newborn baby, in a very similar way to how they managed their role at work. They organise.

Consider the phenomenon that is the Gina Ford system. A structured approach that establishes a regular and repeated pattern into the baby's day – and for many, many thousands of parents works wonders. It's Outlook for mothers. Of course it also happens to deliver some fantastic results for many thousands of new parents, but the similarities between regulated systems of baby care and the structure of the working day are striking, bordering on the spooky.

But working to a daily schedule is just the tip of the iceberg, what has really become an issue for the modern Dad is the role he plays in Bringing Up Baby Ltd. When a friend of mine with a little girl of a year whispered to me in a quiet moment as I was a month or two away from the arrival of my son 'never pack the bag', I was puzzled. He explained that in his experience offering to make sure everything you need for the little one is in the obligatory baby bag ahead of a trip out, is a great thing to do in theory. In practice, however, he assured me that it was doomed to failure, that in the eyes of the mother it would be a well-meaning attempt, but ultimately a big fat nil point, because it wouldn't be packed quite right.

Surely not I thought, surely that's just the lack of sleep talking? But no. Across the land thousands of new fathers are experiencing the same plight; being asked to do more, but never quite coming up to scratch. Whether it's the wrong trousers, the wrong blanket or the wrong type of teat, being a junior partner in the company can be very tough.

Differences of opinion before didn't matter that much really you see; a holiday destination here, a rug there, debate could rage, words could be even be exchanged, but on the whole compromise reached. But this is different, this is life and death.

New Dad: 'I think he's tired.'

New Mum: 'He's not tired, that's a hungry cry.'

New Dad: 'He's probably got a bit of wind.'

New Mum: 'He's just been winded, he's tired.'

New Dad: 'I think he needs a jumper on, it's cold in here.'

New Mum: 'Feel the back of his neck, he's overheating if anything. Are you trying to kill him?'

So the last one has a touch of dramatic licence to it, but you get the picture. Mother knows best, she is all over baby and what baby needs like a rash because she is built to do just that and is with him all day long while you, well you're just guessing. What's a man meant to do?

Seize the day

The answer to that question is simpler than you'd imagine, talk and start talking right now.

There's a chance of course that you might have the most angelic baby ever conceived, you might be independently wealthy or incredibly stealthy and get out of any baby duties by either employing an army of staff or pretending to have a hernia and taking to your bed for six months.

But more likely than not, new and fiendishly testing situations will arise within your relationship at a frequent rate and trying to calmly pause, identify and discuss what is at the heart of them will be your undoubted objective. The only trouble is it will be 3.47am, one of you will be singing 'Hush little baby don't say a word' for the thousandth time while a burning pain starts to spread through your already broken back and the other will be hunting frantically for the gripe water.

But for the next month or two before your baby arrives you've got the opportunity to spend an hour or two at the very least trying to set a few ground rules, to promise each other that no matter what happens love is indeed all around and tolerance will be your watchword. It mightn't make all that much difference in the frantic first few months, but when tiredness seeps through every pore, even one argument avoided will make your pre-birth efforts more than worth it.

....

Words from your fellow man:

Kevin, 50, had two children in his early twenties, followed by two more in his forties, the dirty dog: *I honestly can't remember changing a single nappy when my first two were small. And I'm not some sort of 'Where's my dinner woman' brute by any means – you just didn't get involved back then. My wife gave up work as a matter of course and I expected to and was expected to provide for them all. I worked hard and when I got home from work the kids were bathed and tucked up in bed.*

Second time around it's been totally and utterly different. I've changed nappies, had them screaming on my shoulder at 4am and made bath time my own – I've been totally involved and it's been absolutely fantastic.

I think people forget though just how much attitudes have changed in such a short space of time. You got funny looks and even the odd comment pushing your child in a pram as a bloke just 30 years ago. Now I wander down the street with my nipper in the sling and no one bats an eye lid. It's great but it's a mind-blowing change.

Nick, 35, father of two: *The change to our relationship was huge. I expected it to be much easier. The penny really dropped when I was having to read the instructions of the breast pumping machine (which were in German) at 2am in the morning. That was indicative of what our relationship now revolved around.*

At the beginning my opinion on what to do with our son didn't carry equal weight at all.

My wife was great and I felt like a weekend Dad at times – mostly because I was. In fact that was probably the cause of quite a lot of issues – I come home from work after she'd had a really heavy day with Lucas and I'd throw my tuppence worth in without thinking.

You are very much in the thick of it together and while it was easy to blame each other for lack of sleep we were also focused on the new baby. It's not really your relationship that changes, it's your lives.

Jim, 34, father of one: *We are a partnership, a team, we talk about everything and always did before the baby arrived too. I think we are doing alright, it's a tough job. In some ways we are closer yet further apart, perhaps because there is someone else in the middle.*

Suki, 34, father of one: *You have to get used to doing things differently and obviously you have to plan your lives a lot more than you did before, a lot more. You also have to accept that you are no longer the most important person around, in fact you're not even the second most important person around.*

David, 34, father of one: *I got home from work one day and my wife handed me a leaflet from our local opticians: 'I'm worried', she said 'about your eyes, I think you might be short sighted.' 'Really?' 'Yes, I don't think you can see anything that is below your knees – it's the only explanation I can come up with as to why you constantly walk up the stairs and straight past 20 fucking things that need taking up there.'*

Premature births

It's thought that more than 50,000 babies are born prematurely each year in the UK, which equates to around one in eight deliveries. That's a staggeringly high figure when you give it some thought and it is very much on the increase.

Pre-term is defined as being born before 37 weeks' gestation and in truth the condition is still not well understood with most early births still happening without any clear reason. It's hard to say who will have a premature birth, but it seems you're more likely to if your partner:

> Has given birth early before

> Has had a miscarriage late in pregnancy

> Has had an infection in her birth canal or womb

> Has a weak cervix and tends to open early (our old friend cervical incompetence)

> Has a bleeding placenta

> Is carrying more than one baby (half of all sets of twins and most sets of triplets are born early)

> Is a smoker

It pays to be on the look-out for the very early signs of labour, which include: any type of contraction-like sensation; low, dull backache; pelvic pressure or pain, diarrhoea; vaginal spotting; bleeding; and watery vaginal discharge. As ever if your partner has so much as a scintilla of doubt, get in touch with your doctor or midwife ASAP.

Born survivors

Survival rates for premature babies in developed countries have been creeping up and up in the past 20 years as technology and expertise have moved on. As a rough guide, around 17% of babies born at 23 weeks survive, rising up to 50% at 25 weeks and 90% at 27 weeks.

By the 34th week, it's reckoned that a prematurely born baby has almost the same chance of survival as a full-term baby [31]. The very latest research paints an even more hopeful picture with about 70% of babies born between 22 and 26 weeks' gestation in Sweden now making it past their first birthday with medical intervention [32].

But it's the nature and especially the timing of the medical intervention that remains such a controversial issue. A 2006 report by the Nuffield Council on Bioethics, which provides guidelines around morally difficult medical issues [33], stated that babies born before 22 weeks and six days gestation should not generally be resuscitated and that below 22 weeks no baby should be resuscitated whatsoever. Even between 23 weeks and 23 weeks and six days, there is no legal obligation on doctors to try to save a baby if they judge it to be against the child's best interests, which given the survival rates we have just seen is a real anomaly.

It's a tremendously complex issue, but what's simple to grasp is that having a premature baby today is vastly different from going through the same thing even a decade ago.

Long-term effects

Despite the improved survival rates of premature babies it's clear that many still face a number of challenges both immediately after birth and in later life. In the immediate aftermath of their birth the tiny tots are susceptible to breathing problems due to underdeveloped lungs. They are also at greater risk of cerebral palsy and a number of life-threatening infections. Later on in life there seems to be some evidence that they are more likely to have learning and developmental disabilities.

A recent study [34] analysed the IQ and academic ability of 219 children born extremely premature – before 26 weeks – back in 1995. The children's performance was compared with that of 153 classmates who had all been born after a normal length pregnancy. One in three of the prematurely born children found reading a real effort, while 44%

struggled with maths. These children also scored slightly lower on IQ than their contemporaries.

Keeping the faith

Despite all the worries and anguish that inevitably comes with a premature birth there are plenty of stories to give hope to everyone who goes through one.

Perhaps the most astonishing is that of Amillia Taylor, who was born on 24 October 2006 in Miami at just 21 weeks and six days' gestation. At birth, she was 9 inches long and weighed 10 ounces (0.625 lbs) – so about as long as a pen and no heavier than a can of Coke. Given that the American Academy of Pediatrics state that babies born at less than 23 weeks are not 'viable', she not only cheated nature, but she also cheated the law as well thanks to the fact that in desperation her mother Sonja didn't let on to doctors just how early she was.

Nine days after Sonja showed signs of labour at just 19 weeks, her doctors realised that they couldn't delay the birth any longer and performed a caesarean. Unbelievably Amillia came out breathing without assistance and even made some tiny, tiny attempts to cry. At this, medical staff assumed that she might be 23 weeks old and understandably Sonja didn't put them right, fearing what the consequences could be.

Despite suffering digestive and respiratory problems, as well as a brain haemorrhage, Amillia was discharged from hospital four months later and is now a healthy little girl.

If you go through a premature birth, keep the faith and take heart, not just from Amillia, but also from the fact that Isaac Newton and Winston Churchill were both believed to have been born early too and they made a half decent fist of life didn't they?

The progress report

Month 7 (Baby is 27-31 weeks old)

Your baby

Bad news, this is the last month that your baby can turn a summersault in the womb. He can still kick though and will do so increasingly; probably because he's raging that he hasn't got room to do acrobatics anymore. That's it, no more fooling around now little one, it's time to get ready for the serious stuff.

By the end of this month your baby will measure around 28cm from crown to rump and weigh in at about 1.5kg (3.5lbs), which is starting to sound a bit more like a baby's weight isn't it?

As well as fattening up, your baby is continuing to mature and become more independent, ready for going it alone in a few weeks time. He can now control his own body temperature and his bone marrow has now taken complete responsibility for the making of his red blood cells.

He has also developed a mature breathing pattern by now and the air sacs in his lungs are beginning to get ready for his first breath. Chances are that he will still need initial help in breathing if he arrived now though.

He is now passing urine into the amniotic fluid at the rate of about a pint every day, which seems like a lot of wee for someone so wee. Mind you, now they have fully functioning taste buds on their tongue and inside their cheeks they must surely be starting to realise that the amniotic marketing board may have been over-egging its product's appeal slightly.

Your baby's brain is also starting a growth spurt this month and to squeeze inside its skull it starts to fold over on itself, which is why all of brains take on that weird walnut look.

At about this time your baby's eyelids begin to open too and studies have shown that when a torch is shone against the stomach, the baby may move towards or away from the beam, which when you think about it doesn't prove much really does it, but there you go I thought I'd pass it on.

In all probability though your baby is becoming more sensitive to light, sound, taste and smell.

The colour of your baby's eyes begins to appear around now too, but the real colour won't show until six to nine months after birth, because eye pigmentation needs light exposure to complete its formation – or you could just shine that torch at the bump a lot more to speed things up a bit. I'm joking of course, but you knew that didn't you.

Your partner

It's a big welcome back to utter tiredness for your better half as the third trimester kicks in. It's a state that in truth she, and indeed you, will remain in for the next six or seven years. Fatigue will become like an old, crotchety, short-tempered companion that will never really leave your side for very long. Enjoy.

Apart from that though there are all sorts of exciting anatomical and physiological things going on as your partner prepares for the most complex, overwhelming and at the same time breathtaking thing she will ever do.

She may well be already producing colostrum, the sweet, watery fluid which is less rich than breast milk proper and easier for a baby, so far used to a diet consisting exclusively of amniotic matter, to digest. This is the stuff that will, all being well, provide your baby with his first few meals and it is so packed full of antibodies and nutrients that I'd be here for the rest of my life if I attempted to list them.

It's also hello old friend to needing to go to the loo 250 times a day. As the baby grows and grows it begins to press on your partner's bladder in a big way.

This is also the stage in which the lower back pain that forces pregnant women to stand hand on hip like a Les Dawson character kicks in. A combination of the alteration of her centre of gravity and the slight loosening of the pelvic joints to allow for a baby to pop out are the culprits.

Bump-wise things are getting quite prominent now and it's only a matter of days before someone plucks up the courage to risk the classic not pregnant just fat response and offer her a seat on the bus.

There's a fair chance your partner will be offered an antenatal check at least every two weeks from now until around the 36th week and she can ask about anything that's worrying her. Things such as varicose veins can cause real anxiety at this stage, as can breathlessness, which can occur as her lungs absorb about 20% more oxygen and expel more carbon dioxide with each intake, as she essentially breathes for two.

Finally you may notice your partner's tummy button starting to become stretched and elongated, or even protrude. No matter how it looks, the baby will not – repeat will not – be coming out through the naval, and all will be back to normal after the birth. Just wanted to put your mind at rest on that one.

THE MUST-DOS OF THE MONTH

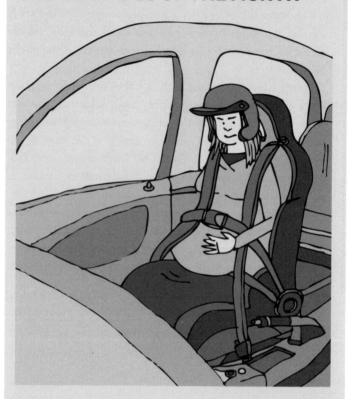

Belt up
If you've not done so already a pregnancy seat belt extension is a very good idea. It essentially means that in the event of an accident, the belt doesn't put pressure on the bump.

Treat her
A pregnancy massage, a pedicure, a manicure, a face mask – booking a little treatment treat for her at this stage when the chances of her reaching her toes to paint them is receding by the second, will go down a storm.

Stroll on

Walking is your friend. It's not only a great way to spend some time together and talk about how you are both feeling, it also means your partner is getting some gentle but invaluable exercise and fresh air.

Give some back up

Back pain is a nightmare at the best of times. Suffering from it when you're pregnant though is as annoying as it is inevitable. That doesn't mean you can't do something to keep your partner's discomfort to a minimum though.

Buying her a pair of low-heeled or flat shoes that don't look they have been stolen from a bowling alley is a good start. Gently encouraging her to sit with a straight back on a hard chair or the floor is smart too, although be prepared to be told occasionally to stop acting like her mother. There are also bump support belts available, which take some of the strain off the back.

If you get one of these under no circumstances refer to it as her truss.

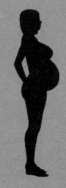

MONTH 8
Last orders please

Everyone knows that pregnancy is nine months long. As soon as you enter the first day of that final month the baby could arrive any day, any second, or at least that's the perceived wisdom.

So what does that make the eighth month then?

Busy, that's what it makes it, very busy.

The reality of the ninth month being a quick hop, skip and a jump to the delivery can be very different of course. For a start you've often got four weeks of the bloody thing to negotiate before full term is reached and even then around one in every five women goes over term and needs to be induced.

But none of that matters, especially when you're having your first baby: nine months is when it's due, so eight months is your last chance to get things sorted before your little family increases in size.

As if to bolster this chronological logic, our old pals the pregnancy hormones bring the nesting instinct to the party, with all its quirks, idiosyncrasies and Hoover-mania. And I'm not just talking about your partner here, as we've seen on the phantom pregnancy front there is increasing evidence that men's hormones lead them a merry dance in the lead up to pregnancy too. So then, eyes down for a frantic four weeks.

You've gotta love a list

If lists weren't invented by men, it was certainly something we would have got round to doing. Lists are a man's best friend; put something down on one and you've as good as done it, or at least as good as stopped having to think about the bloody thing.

There's an awful lot to do this month and even if there wasn't, it seems we are programmed to feel like there is, both socially and hormonally – the eighth month is the pregnancy equivalent of the pre-Christmas rush.

So let's throw ourselves into it and look at what needs to be done, what's the best way to do it and how, among all the hullaballoo, everyone involved can find the time for a good sit down too.

The birth plan

Let's not bugger about, let's get straight in there with the daddy of all lists – the birth plan.

Viewed by many as the chocolate fireguard of the pregnancy process, the birth plan is a way of rationally and calmly telling the people who are caring for your partner what she would like to happen and what she would most certainly not like to happen.

Your partner will of course communicate in no uncertain terms with the health professionals when she is in labour, but the calm and rational bits will go out of the window, along with the doctor's stethoscope if she can get near enough to grab it. So this written plan essentially acts as a letter written by your partner when she was sane. It's surely only a matter of time before boring old paper is replaced by a short movie projected on the wall of the delivery suite for all staff to watch.

'Hello, the fact that you're watching this that means I'm lying on a bed with my legs in the air screaming some fearful obscenities.'

No matter what format it's in though, one thing is for absolute certain about your birth plan: it will always be a work of fiction to a less or greater degree – and so it should be.

Sitting on your couch two months out and writing with a great deal of sincerity and conviction that 'under no circumstances do we want any pain relief outside of gas and air to be administered' is fine. Were your midwife to wave that very piece of paper in your partner's face seven hours into labour as she screamed for every drug known to modern medicine, you'd wish you'd kept your pen in its holster.

But luckily that's not how it works at all. Most smart birth plans are written very carefully like a communiqué at a G8 summit; with certain avenues favoured, but leaving none blocked off.

Given the unpredictable nature of childbirth and the differing ways which people cope with what it throws at them, there's every chance that the midwife may well need to recommend a course of action that is not what either of you had in mind, but one which is in the best interests of your baby.

Writing it

There's no hard-and-fast rules about how to write a birth plan. As you can imagine the web is awash with print out and fill in templates, but as this is such a personal document you may find that you use these as just a guide and essentially go it alone.

Some people structure them chronologically: early stages, transition, delivery etc; others write theirs issue by issue: pain relief, favoured positions, feeding the baby. Whichever way your partner prefers to tackle it, it's an idea to bear these three points in mind:

> Make sure it's no more than one page in length. It has been scientifically proven that no one has read anything longer than one side of A4 since 1981.

> Do your research beforehand – don't mix up an episiotomy with a cup of sweet tea.

> Be direct, but be nice.

Is it worth it?

Good question.

Some say that the best thing you can do with your birth plan when you arrive at hospital is to keep it in the bag. Walking into such a fluid and unpredictable situation with a semi-rigid set of demands doesn't help anyone, they say. If you brandish it too lustily there's also the fear that it could even mark you out as a patient from hell, although that theory does the medical staff who will be on hand a massive disservice in my opinion. Even worse though, it could act as a stick to beat yourselves with, a record of the control you'd like to have in one of the most uncontrolled environments you'll ever find yourselves in.

On the other side of the coin there's no doubt at all that the very act of thinking about and writing the birth plan together as a couple, means that you both focus on the potential issues that may arise at a time when you can think clearly and at least go some way to addressing them mentally. For that reason alone it's got to be a list worth making.

....

Words from your fellow man:

Stuart, 37, father of two: *Our birth plan said gas and air and epidural as a very last resort. Within half an hour with gas and air my partner was begging for the epidural. The birth plan for your first baby isn't based on any kind of reality. It's like trying to imagine how you'd feel taking a penalty in the World Cup Final while sitting in your armchair with a beer in your hand.*

Peter, 33, father of one: *We had planned for a water birth but as things went really quickly we didn't have time to run the bath. Ironically I have been plagued with shit baths all my life that only ever dribble out water from the taps, but I did expect the NHS to have got round this problem. We took lots of CDs and candles as well but they are still in a plastic bag in the boot of the car.*

Levi, 36, father of two: *We did pretty much stick to our birth plan, although our baby did get stuck upside down for five hours in my wife's nether regions. Otherwise it went like clockwork.*

The hospital bag

There's nothing like the sight of a fully packed bag sitting quietly, expectantly, in the corner of the bedroom, to remind you that at some point soon everything you've been reading about, talking about and thinking about for months, will begin to happen.

In many ways, though, the hospital bag has also become a sign of the times: a pregnancy icon, a window into our world of gadgetry and deep-seated fear of missing a trick – if only, if only, we'd brought the colander.

But really it's just a bag of stuff you might need but probably won't use and more often than not your departure for the hospital isn't anywhere near as Hollywood as you are led to believe it will be. The process of labour itself is also often such a long, drawn out business that you'll be able to knit your partner a new cardigan should you have left the blue one at home. But as ever with pregnancy you never know.

So what do you really need to take then – the potential list is endless, although I'd leave the dog at home if you can. I've tried to cut out as many of the pointless suggestions that get made – there are lists that recommended taking a pack of cards for instance in case things get a bit dull. The chances of your partner wanting to play a few hands of knockout while in labour are staggeringly remote, unlike the chances of you being served up a volley of abuse for suggesting it.

If you don't understand fully what a few of these things are yet, don't worry, Month 9 is about to give you a run down on all the runners and riders in the delivery room stakes.

For your partner

> The birth plan – seeing as you've spent all that time on it, it would be a shame to leave it on the kitchen table. You could even make multiple copies and start handing them out from the car park onwards to make sure you don't miss out anybody. Or not.

> Medical notes of your partner's health and pregnancy to date.

> Nightdress or pyjamas, dressing gown, slippers, socks – fair enough.

> An old nightdress or T shirt to wear in labour – things could get a bit messy you see.

> Lip balm – sounds ludicrous, but dry and chapped lips after hours of labour is all she'll need.

> Books and magazines – in case of an elongated early labour.

> TENS (transcutaneous nerve stimulation) pain relief machine, if you are planning to use one (more about this on p 205).

> Toiletries – complete range of.

> Music – iPod and speakers or CDs if the hospital has its own system (some hospitals don't let you plug in your own equipment, on the off chance that it shorts the whole place and causes the death of hundreds of people; which for the sake of a Coldplay album would be a very high price to pay indeed).

> Breastfeeding kit – bras, pads, nipple cream, etc, if you plan to give it a go.

> Maternity pads – as I said earlier, things can get a bit messy.

> Old, cheap or disposable knickers – ditto.

> Going home clothes – not quite time for the skinny jeans yet mind you, she will feel like she did at about the six month mark.

> Snacks and drinks – low fat, high carb fare is what's usually on the menu. In truth many women try to load up in the early stages and then can't face a thing until the job is done when they will attempt to eat the midwife's arm. Plenty of fluid is essential.

For yourself

> Water spray – this enables you to carry out one of your traditional and relatively useful labour tasks – trying to keep your partner cool and (relatively) refreshed while she's in labour. Practise your nozzle skills before the big day but don't pick up the Windolene by mistake.

> Digital camera or camcorder – some hospital staff can be funny about you taking pictures; but this is the biggest day of your lives so distract them by pretending to spot a foot-long MRSA bacterium under the bed and snap away at your beautiful new arrival and the wonder woman who brought him into the world.

> Address book/list of phone numbers – you'll want to spread the news ASAP so have what you need to hand to do just that. A fair bit of change is also a smart move as most hospitals hate mobile phones with a passion and you may not want to wander too far from your new family to be able to use one.

> Snacks and drinks – you need to keep your strength up too, tiger. Don't go mad though, the sight of you tucking into a three-course meal with coffee and mints to finish will not go down well with a certain person in the room. Also take real care not to take stuff that's too stinky – I'm not sure if anyone has ever tried to eat a Peperami in front of a labouring woman, but if they have I'm hoping it's on YouTube.

> Bribes – a lot of people send flowers to the midwives after the birth, but a bag of Revels 'to keep the team's strength up' before it all kicks off could pay big dividends when your midwife's shift is about to finish and she's wondering whether to clock off or stick in there.

For the baby

> Baby blanket – to wrap the little mite up in as you take him into the big wide world for the very first time.

> Nappies – the hospital might provide a few, but best to have your own too.

> Socks or booties – bless. Socks on his hands will also

prevent him scratching himself with the sharp little nails he may be born with.

> Hat – for his little bonce.

> Baby grows in XXS, XS and S – who knows how big he's going to be.

> Muslins – let the sick fest begin.

> Infant car seat – not going to fit in the bag this one obviously, but learning how to fit this tricky beast in the car takes a fair bit of time and patience and is best done out of earshot of the midwife. She may not want to entrust a newborn baby to a man who is repeatedly calling a seatbelt a little bastard.

Even with some of the sillier suggestions not making it through the net – such as pen and paper to take notes with (a sure fire way to make the medical staff feel like they are on the maternity equivalent of Masterchef) – it's still a shed load of stuff. Let's just all take a moment to be grateful that Ryanair haven't yet taken to running hospitals shall we – the excess baggage costs would be enormous.

Getting to the hospital

Not technically a list but the chances are you will become strangely obsessed with the various routes you can take to a hospital you know well and have been past many times before. Don't be alarmed, it's perfectly normal. You may even go a stage further and do the journey at eight or nine different times of the day or night and plot a chart of the best route for each hour. That's not so normal.

But hey, this is a big deal and driving your pregnant partner to the hospital is one of the traditional, cast iron father-to-be jobs of all time, so why not get serious on its ass? Besides, it's worth doing a bit of preparation to avoid being stuck at a set of temporary traffic lights for 20 minutes with a passenger who would happily wring your neck should she be able to get off the back seat to reach.

If you've not been to a hospital for a few years allow me to also tell you about a major change you may not be familiar with – the revenue generated by hospital car parks now makes up just under 75% of the entire gross national product of the UK. Or at least that's what it feels like. Take change, take cash, take cards and take gold. If you're in for a long labour you'll need all of them in vast quantities.

One other tiny thing to bear in mind while we are on the transport front, is that as your partner has probably chauffeured you around half pissed for the past eight months, it wouldn't look great if you had to drive her in after having three and half large glasses of merlot. You'll have more than enough on your plate during that journey without hoping beyond hope that a traffic copper doesn't pull you over and take you off the road there and then.

Persona non driva

So what if you don't drive, what are your options?

Calling an ambulance is frowned upon because labour is not classed as an emergency, even though with your first baby it will feel like the most emergencified of all the emergencies you have ever found yourself in. If you do call out one, the chances are that it will take you to the nearest maternity ward rather than the one you are booked in at. If in doubt, always ring the delivery suite at your hospital first and speak to the midwife who will tell you the best course of action to take.

So for most people calling a taxi is the main option open to them. Stories abound of taxi firms refusing to take labouring women in case their car seats take a hammering, so a ring round beforehand to check who is OK to do the job is a smart move.

Oh and give the bendy bus a miss.

Nesting

Your partner is going to start getting very tired this month, very tired indeed. As the baby gets heavier, her energy levels will drain away as the day wears on and the chances of her making it to the end of the evening news will start to dwindle dramatically.

Unless there is decorating to be done of course; or cleaning; or washing all the baby clothes for the second time to get that new smell out of them; or hoovering; or rearranging the stuff in the attic in case the newborn manages to open the hatch, pull down the tricky ladder thing, climb up and become horribly bewildered by the distinct lack of order up there. Tiredness won't affect any of those things.

Welcome to the world of the nesting instinct, where Mother Nature turns pregnant women into frenzied cleaning machines ahead of the new arrival.

As well as often being amusing and sometimes bizarre – some women, rendered so immobile by the sheer size of their bump, have been known to sit in the middle of the floor with the longest vacuum extension they can muster sucking up dust from as wide a radius as they can stretch to – there is something incredibly humbling about being around a nesting woman.

Nesting essentially brings us down from our self-constructed plinth as a super species and acts as yet another reminder, should we need one, that we are really just monkeys with hats on. I say we, because the urge to nest towards the end of pregnancy doesn't just affect women, you can get caught up in the hormonal house cleaning too – you clucky old thing you.

What's the cause?

Prolactin (which is responsible for, among other things, lactation and orgasms and increases in both men and women during pregnancy) is reckoned to be the biggest culprit. Tests on animals show that as nesting and nurturing behaviours in both males and females increase the more prolactin is present.

In fact, so potent is prolactin, on occasion it's not only been nesting and nurturing that it has brought on in males. A Scottish goat named Claymore who is reported to have had an extraordinarily high prolactin level actually started to produce milk. Indeed, so taken was he by the taste of his own milk, that he would often 'nurse himself' – which is one of the most disturbing phrases I've ever had the misfortune to write.

As filthy old Claymore demonstrates, prolactin is one powerful substance and if it can get a billy goat to breastfeed, turning you and your partner into cleaning freaks is no sweat.

How bad can it get?

Pretty bad. Here's a smattering of what could happen:

> Throwing away almost anything, because if it's not new, it's a potential death trap

> Taking apart door knobs and cupboard handles to not only clean inside, but also disinfect the very screws which hold them together

> Adopting the toothbrush as the primary cleaning implement of the household

> Organising kitchen cupboards into package size or alphabetical order depending on what day it is

> Folding and refolding the baby's clothes until they no longer look brand new; which can then invoke the first point on this list

Despite bringing on some pretty irrational behaviour, the only real area to keep your eye on in terms of your partner's nesting instinct is decorating. Climbing ladders and painting aren't the smartest things for a pregnant woman to do, given what a fall could mean and the potential damage that paint fumes can do. By far the safest option is for her to place herself in a comfy chair and creatively direct the whole project as you do the donkey work.

Stopping work

Choosing when to stop work towards the end of the pregnancy can be a very tricky decision for your partner. Some women, imagining that they will want to work until the very last second, find themselves dragging their weary bones on public transport and up office stairs wishing that they hadn't been quite so gung-ho early on. Others, who have given themselves plenty of time off ahead of the big day, can find themselves bored and marooned at home with hour after hour to think about what awaits them on the big day.

It's a hard one to judge and everyone is different, but what's for certain is that whether or not your partner continues to work through to the final knockings, taking it easy as things literally come to a head is a must.

The whole working during pregnancy debate is a thorny one and some studies [35] have claimed that pregnant women who work past the recommended time are up to five times more likely to have the condition of increased blood pressure during pregnancy (including pre-eclampsia) – the inference being that high stress at work causes high blood pressure, which in pregnant women can be deadly.

Whatever the medical facts might be, flexibility is king if your partner is lucky enough to work somewhere that will play ball. Missing the morning rush hour, working from home or trying to avoid the jobs that wind everyone up are all well worth doing at this stage of the game.

If none of them are possible no one but no one is going to question an almost full term woman having a sickie or two – although if anyone asks, remember it wasn't me who suggested that.

The progress report

Month 8 (Baby is 32-35 weeks old)

Your baby

Your baby's main preoccupation at the moment is trying to get himself settled into a head-down position and adjust to the increasing lack of space in the hitherto roomy womb. Once they have found the slot, some babies do decide to turn back round again, although attempted escape at this stage is futile.

By the end of this month the average baby weighs in at around 51/4lbs and is a touch over 18 inches long crown to rump. Because of the nice deposits of fat he is building up, his skin is now a pleasing pink colour rather than a worrying red.

The baby's eyes are now fully functioning and he can focus and blink and as for his ears, it's safe to say that his hearing is better than yours now. Finger and toenails are also fully formed and some babies will even have a full head of hair at this stage, while others might just have a few wisps.

The lungs are still developing though, but even they will be the real deal very soon indeed.

If your baby is a boy his testicles should have dropped from his abdomen into his scrotum. In some cases though one or both testicles won't move into position until after birth and in two-thirds of these babies, the condition corrects itself by the time of their first birthday. Which seems a long time to wait doesn't it?

The baby's skull is still pliable to help him ease out of the narrow birth canal, but all his other bones are hardening, a fact your partner may become well aware of as elbows, feet or even the head itself can start to protrude from her stomach at this point – making you think of, but never mention, the scene from *Alien* where John Hurt has a very bad case of tummy trouble.

Your partner

Antenatal checks will almost certainly be more regular now as blood pressure, urine and the baby's position are kept under a close eye. The level of all-round discomfort felt by your partner also increases this month on a lot of fronts.

Thanks to a pregnancy hormone fantastically called relaxin, your partner's pelvic joints expand and therefore unsurprisingly ache in preparation for birth. There's also more discomfort to be had as the ever-expanding baby forces the womb against your partner's lower ribs, as well as the abdomen, often becoming so stretched that her navel sticks outwards instead of inwards.

She may also notice that her feet and ankles are pretty swollen by the end of the day thanks to water retention.

The following piece of knowledge will almost certainly get you a glare if not something thrown at you, but drinking lots of water actually reduces water retention. Your partner's body and indeed the baby, need plenty of fluids at this point so rather than doing what seems logical and reducing the amount of water she takes in, she needs to increase her intake. Duck.

However, if she suddenly feels swollen or puffy in her hands or face, you should contact your doctor as this may be an indication of pre-eclampsia (p 261).

To top things off nicely, her nipples will also be starting to enlarge and her breasts become heavier; and oh yes, Braxton Hicks contractions (see p 110) can be full on at this stage too, making all concerned very jumpy for the 30 seconds or so they tend to last.

As far as rays of sunshine go, they are few and far between. If the baby has already moved into the head down position, your partner's breathing may become a little easier and indigestion should start to improve; which is something isn't it?

Your partner may also have some fantastically vivid dreams at the moment too. Although, given that they are primarily driven by the thoughts that almost fully formed baby is moving around inside her and she is about to experience childbirth, painting them as light relief may be stretching things a little.

Carpal tunnel syndrome

This annoying late pregnancy complaint deserves to be looked at in a little more detail. Carpal tunnel syndrome (CTS) is a medical condition in which a nerve in the wrist is compressed, leading to numbness, muscle weakness and pain in the hand.

Symptoms are often worse at night and guess what, pregnant women are highly susceptible to it as weight gain and swelling are also contributory factors. Although not all pregnant women suffer from it, it's estimated that between 20% and 60% do, which is a hell of a lot considering the relatively low profile the condition still has.

For most women who do experience it, CTS is generally mild and temporary, disappearing soon after the baby is born, but for others it can be a debilitating and severe problem which can last well into the baby's first year.

A weakened grip, numbness, pain and a burning sensation around the thumb and fingers can combine to make CTS a nightmare for some mothers-to-be and if it does last post pregnancy, it can seriously hamper their ability to lift and carry their newborn.

Flexing wrists and fingers regularly throughout the day is said to help by some and make matters worse by others, so wrist splints worn at night are often the only treatment of any worth. These keep your wrists in a position that provides space in the offending area and eases the problem.

Month 8 isn't much fun for your poor partner is it? Not long now though (although again that's something to be thought but rarely said).

THE MUST-DOS OF THE MONTH

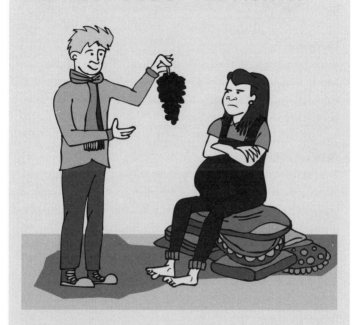

Ring the changes

Haemorrhoids, an ugly looking word for an ugly complaint. If your partner is suffering on the pile front, buy in a job lot of witch hazel – which is a good natural remedy – and offer to apply it regularly. It's the least you can do.

Clocking off

Whether your partner is ecstatic to be finishing work or nervous about putting her hard-fought for career behind her, psychologically it's a big moment and one that does signal the end of one era and the beginning of another.

Make a fuss of her and although you'll be hoarding any spare holiday you have for when the baby is born, taking a day off to spend at home with her after she's jacked in the job is a nice gesture that will almost certainly be appreciated.

Footloose
You've not got long until you are parents. If your partner can handle it make the most of your last few weeks of no-babysitter-required freedom. Eat out, go to the cinema, see friends, and lie in; but not necessarily in that order.

Blowing raspberries
The raspberry leaf contains something called a uterine tonic and, taken daily in the final weeks of pregnancy, it could well help to prepare the uterine muscles for labour and maybe even make the process ever so slightly less painful. In an Australian study [36] 192 first-time mums were given either a 1.2g raspberry leaf tablet or a placebo twice a day from 32 weeks onwards. The lucky ones who were given the real deal were found to have a shorter second stage of labour – which as you are about to read about is the pushing phase – and a significantly lower rate of forceps delivery – 19.3% versus 30.4% in those given placebo. It's fair to say that this was a pretty small study and hardly what you could class as conclusive proof – but it's got to be worth a shot hasn't it?

It's best to start with one cup of raspberry leaf tea a day or one tablet and build up gradually as the due date nears to a maximum of four cups of tea or tablets daily. Your partner can take the tea during labour as well if she's up to it. To the health food shop with you.

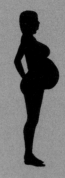

MONTH 9
It's show time

Waiting for curtain up

So here we are, you've made it to the ninth month and all you need to do now is take your seats and the performance will start shortly. Trouble is, as with all the months you tend to come across these days, this bugger is four weeks long, with each day of each week needing to be negotiated individually.

As for the due date you've been given, it's best not to get fixated on it, as only a miserly 5% of babies arrive bang on the money. Out of the remaining 95%, three in every 10 arrive early and seven in 10 late. So the odds are that your partner has still got a fair bit of incubating to do yet – even as much as six weeks more from the start of this month in fact, which is pretty much the longest the medical profession in the UK will let you wait before they deem the placenta too old and inefficient to properly nourish the baby any longer.

All that of course presupposes that the due date itself is based on sound medical and mathematical principles. Which it isn't.

Most estimated due dates are calculated using a formula devised by a German obstetrician named Franz Naegele in the 1850s. The rule estimates the date from the first day of the woman's last menstrual period by adding a year, subtracting three months and adding seven days to that date. This Johnny Ball-like equation roughly works the average normal human pregnancy out to last around 280 days, or 40 weeks, from the date of fertilisation.

Among the many inconsistencies of this outdated method is that it relies on the notion that in 19th-century Deutschland women evidently ovulated on the 14th day of a 28-day cycle without fail or they would be locked in the woodshed to think about what they had done.

Another of its drawbacks is that it relies on each month having 30.4 days in it exactly – so get pregnant in May, or God forbid in a leap year, and your due date stands a very good chance of being well out.

Basically, it's a bloody rubbish system that almost always gives us due dates that are too early. But we just haven't got round to replacing it yet, what with global warming to sort out and the effort we all had to put in to get Wispas back on the shelves.

All of which means that before you get to the main event, there's a good chance you'll have to get through another month of being pregnant – which is a pain in the arse for you and a pain absolutely everywhere for your poor partner. So let's quickly zip through what's what in Month 9 before it all kicks off.

The progress report

Month 9 (Baby is 36-40 weeks old)

Your baby

Your baby is considered full term at 37 weeks, meaning that he can be born any day. If labour starts now no effort will be made to delay it; it's for real.

On average your baby will measure about 37–38cm from crown to rump, with a total length of about 48cm, but of course as we already know, all of the little bubbas are different.

The final pieces of the baby's anatomical jigsaw are put into place this month: the central nervous system is all but fully wired, the digestive system is complete and his lungs mature to full capacity leaving him ready to breathe his first ever breath.

His skin is smooth and soft as a baby's bottom, especially his bottom, and there is still the odd dollop of the cream cheese substitute vernix around, mostly on his back to help his passage down the birth canal.

His fingernails are probably long too due to him not being able to find his tiny nail clippers in there – something you will come to empathise with shortly – and he may well have already scratched his face, bless him.

Most of your baby's lanugo – the fine downy hair that's covered it for a good portion of the pregnancy so far – has now been shed. Delightfully he will now swallow the lot along with other secretions, and store them in his bowels ready to form his first poo – a tacky, post-Guinness-drinking-session-like stool called meconium.

All in all after nine remarkable months of growth the goose is cooked – transformed from a bag of cells to a little person – and it's heading your way.

Your partner

The poor, poor woman – even though there's only weeks, even days left to go, time may well feel like it's standing still as she wrestles with her sheer size. Posture-wise she could well find herself making up for the extra weight out front by leaning backwards hands on the back of her hips in classic *Rising Damp* style.

Such is the change in her centre of gravity she could also find herself bumping into things or losing balance, so one of your many jobs this month is to be a helping hand where needed.

In most first-time mothers, the baby's head drops down or engages into the pelvis at about 36 weeks – although in subsequent pregnancies it's normal for your baby to get cocky and not to engage until the last minute.

The most important thing for your partner to do at this stage is to sleep and rest. The most difficult thing for your partner to do at this stage is sleep and rest.

Those jolly japers, the Braxton Hicks contractions, will still be knocking around too, scaring the bejesus out of her, although she's probably an expert at spotting their phoney baloney twinges by now. If they become painful though, then it's time to take notice.

Excitement, nervousness and even fear can be swirling around in pretty significant measure as the clock ticks down. Some women even experience depression in late pregnancy, because of lack of sleep and a deep, deep desire for the baby to be outside rather than in. Combine with trepidation to produce an overwhelming cocktail. It's pretty rare but keep an eye out for it and keep talking.

Another uncommon thing to keep a little watch out for is the onset of severe itchiness in your partner. This can be a sign of a serious liver problem called obstetric cholestasis. If this is the case the itchiness will be very widespread and often includes itching of the hands and feet. It may also be accompanied by nausea, vomiting, loss of appetite, fatigue, pale-coloured stools and jaundice.

Make an appointment with your doctor or midwife if you are worried.

Something not to be too concerned about is if your partner's weight plateau's now – a few women even lose weight in the last week or so before the birth. This barely needs saying, but the main issue in Month 9 is that your partner's stomach is being crushed by a great big baby – she is going to be one uncomfortable soon-to-be momma and it's down to you to keep her if not happy, then at least on the right side of volcanic.

THE MUST-DOS OF THE MONTH

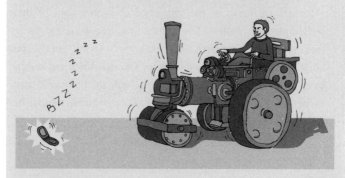

Will you fuck off

Get into the habit early of politely telling friends and family that you'll let them know as soon as something happens, rather than them needing ask.

It's a long enough month without having to field daily requests asking for 'any news' and although reading this you may think me a miserable bastard and that you will never react to people's interest with anything other than unbridled gratitude – I promise eventually it will annoy you to the very core of your being.

Cook up a storm

When your baby arrives home you'll be all over the place for a few weeks as the normalities of everyday life, such as eating and sleeping, get hijacked by the new person in the nappy.

While you can't really prepare for the sleep deprivation, you can make moves to ensure you and your partner (who will be recovering from a major trauma and even major surgery if she's had a caesarean section and may also be breastfeeding and needing to keep her food intake up) aren't reduced to consoling yourselves that the corn on the cob in the KFC bucket you've just bought at least constitutes one of your five a day.

Fill the freezer with frozen shepherd's pies, lasagnes, (mild) chillies – whatever nutritious comfort foods you fancy in fact, and you'll be glad to call on this scrumptious stockpile when times get tough.

Chill
Sounds obvious, but the pair of you should do your best to relax as much as possible this month.

Walking remains a great option if your partner's up for it and the movement is even thought to bring on labour. Or if something less strenuous is in order go the pictures or join a postal DVD club and make every night movie night – no birth DVDs though eh.

As far as you're concerned you could squeeze a last game of golf in – not last game forever, but last for a while, or go to a match. Or – my personal recommendation is stay in bed as much as you can and savour the knowledge that you could get up if you wanted to – but crucially you don't have to.

Coiled spring
Just in case you've forgotten, your partner could go into labour at any second so keep your mobile on, the car full of petrol and your bloodstream free of too much alcohol so you can drive the thing. And relax.

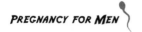
The birth plot - what's meant to happen

You are about to play a part in one of the biggest and most dramatic scenes of your entire life. It'll have the lot: tension, agony, despair and elation – and although you'll be familiar with the general thrust of the story, this is no re-run; this will be unique to you and your partner, never to be forgotten.

Before we get on to who the main players are and how the action might unfold, it's worth taking a quick look at the mechanics of how a birth works, at what the script says should actually happen.

Much like the act of conception, childbirth is one of those things that as men we profess to fully understand, but when it comes to the details we start to mumble and jibber like fools. A bit like how a car engine actually works, or why, despite the very best of intentions, not a single man has found the item he was looking for in a drawer since 1907.

So here's a straight biological run down of what it takes to turn a bump into a baby before we go on to look at what's likely to actually happen when you add emotion, a room full of people, bucketfuls of hormones and not a little pain into the mix.

The stages of labour

According to the textbooks labour moves forward in three clear stages:

The first stage
During the first stage, contractions will gradually open up the neck of the cervix. This stage is itself split into three sections – early labour, active labour and the transitional phase.

Early labour: Sometimes referred to as the latent phase, early labour sees the cervix soften, open and widen thanks to various chemicals acting on it. This process is to allow the baby to pass through it and down into the birth canal before it sees the light at the end of the tunnel and makes a break for freedom. The cervix will go from being tightly closed to about 3cm or 4cm open or dilated – once this happens active labour has started.

Active labour: At this point contractions usually become longer, more frequent and often more painful – the cervix is now opening from 3cm or 4cm to the magic 10cm needed. The contractions themselves could come as often as every three to four minutes and last 60–90 seconds at this stage, or they can even be as frequent as five in a 10-minute period.

Transition: The transitional phase is when your partner moves from the first to the second, pushing, stage. It's often talked about as the period when the cervix moves from 8cm dilated to the full 10cm – the hard yards.

While contractions may be less frequent during this phase, they can be much stronger and longer and can even come in a double wave, with the fading away of one being overtaken by the rise of the next.

It's quite common for your partner's waters to break just before or during transition. During pregnancy the baby is protected and cushioned inside the uterus in a bag full of amniotic fluid. When the bag tears and fluid leaks out, it is the waters breaking. Most women's waters break towards the end of the first stage of labour, but for about 10% of women the waters break before labour starts (in this situation a doctor or midwife should always be seen to reduce the risk of infection) and for the remaining 2%, the waters break before they are 37 weeks' pregnant. The amount of fluid that comes out will vary from a discreet trickle to a take-cover tidal wave.

After such an intense phase you, your baby and especially your partner will need a rest, and nature often provides this through a short lull in the contractions before the big push.

In terms of the length of this first phase for women carrying their first baby, the average rate of cervical dilation is 1cm per hour in active labour (ie from around 3cms dilated onwards). There are huge variations in labour length but the average length of time for the cervix to dilate completely is 9.7 hours. Durations longer than 24.7 hours are considered prolonged – which you'd hope they would be!

The second stage
Once your partner has reached this point she is ready to push your baby out through the birth canal – a distance of around 9 inches – and into the world. She'll feel the pressure of the baby's head between her legs and with each contraction will come a strong urge to push.

With every push, the baby will move gradually through the pelvis a little until the almost-mother starts to feel a stinging sensation – which is caused by the opening of the vagina starting to stretch around the head. Once the midwife can see the baby's head she may ask your partner to stop pushing and take short breaths for the next couple of contractions to help ensure that the baby is born slowly to reduce the likelihood of tearing occurring or the need for a cut called an episiotomy (see p 250) to be made to allow the baby through.

A few more pushes, and the baby is born. The average length of the second phase for first-time Mums is between one and two hours.

The third stage
Once the baby is born, the third stage begins. A new batch of contractions, thankfully weaker this time, will start up again and gradually force the placenta away from the wall of the uterus.

With the aid of the odd push, the placenta, with the membranes of the empty bag of waters attached, will drop out through the vagina. In many hospitals, new mothers are routinely give an injection that makes the placenta come out without the need for any pushing.

The midwife will then examine the placenta and membranes to make sure that nothing has been left behind and check your partner's abdomen to ensure that her uterus is contracting to stop the bleeding caused by the placenta coming away.

The cast list

Alright, so now we know the basic plan: slowly open the heavy, stiff and rusty hanger doors, push the enormous aircraft through them, before making sure you remember to drag out the parachute it's pulling behind it too.

But very few births run anywhere nearly as smoothly as a quick one, two, three and out you pop – especially when the baby is the woman's first.

One of the many reasons why childbirth is so unpredictable is that the process of giving birth that we have adopted tends to involve an awful lot more people than you'd imagine. So before we look at what's *likely* to happen rather than what *should* happen, let's just find out who's who on the delivery cast list for the average hospital birth.

The mother-to-be: If you're not recognising her at this stage you really are in deep trouble – or possibly the wrong delivery room. The absolute star of the show – until she gets upstaged in the final scene by a devastatingly endearing child actor. Although prone to foul-mouthed outbursts, she is a truly committed and focused performer – grappling with the job in hand with such gusto and courage that no one can take their eyes off her.

Midwife: One of life's natural supporting actors – attentive, caring and knowledgeable, although not beyond delivering a forceful word or two should the situation require it. Increasingly though there are tragic occasions where time and shift patterns get the better of these devoted helpers and they have to exit stage right before the dramatic final scene.

Second midwife: A notoriously tricky role. Entering the fray part-way through, she often has to gain trust and respect in double quick time and can find herself on the receiving end of one of the leading lady's legendary tirades. Despite these initial tensions most understudy midwives turn out to be good eggs in the end, but some are condemned to remain peripheral figures, never escaping the lateness at which they joined the performance.

Doctor: Often cast as the portent of doom, this white-coated willow-the-wisp makes rare and fleeting visits to check on progress – until something is amiss, when they swing into action and take charge of proceedings, often putting noses out of joint in the process.

Student doctor: Green behind the gills but eager to learn, these pasty faced trainees often pop up nowadays. Hovering over the midwife's shoulder it takes all their might to keep the air of doctorly superiority that is being ingrained in them under wraps. Can occasionally be heard to mutter, 'That's that done, geriatrics next', once the show is over.

Doula/birthing partner: A relative newcomer on the scene, these guardian angels exist for one reason only: to act as the experienced eyes and ears for the mother as she throws herself headlong into her role. Not for the faint-hearted, this is a part often played by those with a natural propensity to speak up rather than take their own counsel. Can be a generator of flying sparks.

Baby: A scene stealer is born. Despite only making the briefest of appearances towards the very end of proceedings, this tiny totem manages to make his presence very much felt, despite spending the majority of his time out of view.

And finally...

The father-to-be: A well-intentioned but peripheral figure present throughout but never managing to establish a clear role. Often gives off a self-conscious air of being neither useful nor an ornament.

Or so popular culture would lead us to believe. The panicking and ineffectual father flapping around the delivery room, water spray in one hand, roast beef sandwich in the other, has become a comedy staple. Yet figures put the percentage of men attending the birth of their children in the UK at somewhere between 90% and 98% – which is a staggering figure when you consider that 50 years ago the practice was all but unheard of.

The debate rages about the positive and negative effects, on both the mother and the father, that being there brings; the main negative cited being that labour can be longer, more painful and more complicated because she senses his anxiety and becomes nervous herself. It's an interesting argument and one which very quickly arrives at the point that says exclusively female birth environments (including no male doctors etc.) are the least likely to add to the labouring woman's troubles [37].

Chances are though you are going to be there, so assuming you can stop yourself screaming 'Blood, blood, I can see blood!', let's look at the crucial role you can play in supporting your partner.

First things first, no one in that room, not the doctor, not the midwife, not the doula, knows your partner better than you do. If you've been to antenatal classes together and talked about what her fears and expectations are, you are perfectly placed to be her advocate, the person who can speak up when you feel the need.

That's easier said than done for sure. A delivery room full of medical professionals can be a very intimidating place, a factor which is behind the rise in popularity of professional birth partners and doulas who have experience of intervening in those pressure cooker situations.

But you're not just there to be a thorn in the side of the midwives. One study showed that fathers are five times more likely to touch their partner during labour and delivery than other support figures; and the women rated the fathers' presence more helpful than that of the nurses [38].

Providing you keep your emotions in check, you can bring calm and comfort to your partner in a way that no one else can. Just being there can often be enough. It's a tough job of course, you'll get cursed and worse, but let's face it, you'd take sitting next to the bed over being the one on it any day of the week wouldn't you?

Let's not get ahead of ourselves though, we're about to find out what having a baby is really like from the initial faint twinge to first family cuddle.

Action!

So far we know what's meant to happen and we know who's meant to be there – but how do things tend to pan out? What's having a baby really like?

Are we nearly there yet?

For many years, it was believed that the mother's body was responsible for starting labour, but research now points to the baby himself as the one to kick the whole thing off by pressing the hormonal eject button and sending a message to his Mum to get a move on.

One theory is that the baby's lungs secrete an enzyme when they are fully developed which triggers contractions, another is that glands near the baby's kidneys do the deed and expel a hormone that starts things moving.

Whatever starts it, one of the most curious things about childbirth is that for something so profound, so dramatically life-changing, it almost always starts with more of a whimper than a bang.

In fact, it's next to impossible to be absolutely sure in the very early stages whether this is the start of it all, or just a bit of backache. To add to the frustration, when you ask someone in the know *how* you'll know, they just say with a smile, 'Don't worry, you'll *know*!' Just writing that has brought all the annoyance that phrase conjures up flooding back.

The only other time in my life I remember being given such wet advice was when learning to drive.

Me: 'When do you change gear?'

Instructor: 'You'll know.'

Me: 'No, I don't know, how will I know when to change gear?'

Instructor: 'Don't worry, you'll just know.'

Me: 'I won't, I'm telling you, I don't know.'

Instructor: 'You'll know, the car will tell you, you'll just know.'

CRASH

What's even more annoying was that my driving instructor was right of course – drunk but right – and so it is with the onset of labour. You, or rather your partner, will just know when labour has started because she will have some or all of the symptoms listed below.

> Your partner could experience lower back or abdominal pain that persists and is often accompanied by a crampy premenstrual-type feeling.

> Some women get diarrhoea-like symptoms in early labour as the body has a good old clear out ready to give birth.

> A brownish or blood-tinged mucus discharge called the bloody show comes away (please avoid using the line about making a bloody show of yourself, no matter how tempting – now really isn't the time). This is the mucus plug that blocks the cervix, helps to keep the baby in and infection out – and it's not there any more! Get the bag, we're off to the hospital! Not so fast, mucus man – this could be a sign that labour is imminent, or it could be several days away. Bugger. Either way though it is a sign that things are moving along nicely.

PREGNANCY FOR MEN

> Painful contractions that occur at regular but shortening intervals and become longer and stronger – bit of a giveaway that one.

Some or all of the above may happen in the early stages, but don't expect fireworks to go off when labour actually starts, the whole thing is much more of a fluid process than the stage 1, 2 and 3 model would suggest.

It's official

Once your partner's body is telling her unequivocally that she is in labour, when the pains she's feeling are becoming longer, stronger and more frequent, you are on your way. It's a very strange time in many ways, this event that you have been waiting for every day for nine months has finally started to happen and your natural reaction is to call in international rescue, but instead you'll probably just put the kettle on.

Many women describe this early pain as feeling like a bad period pain cramp that reaches a peak, eases off and returns at regular intervals. The contractions may only last about 20 seconds and be 15–20 minutes apart when they first start, or they could start off much stronger and closer together. Because first labours are usually at least 12 hours long it's probably best not to go to hospital too soon. Your partner will be infinitely more relaxed at home than she will in hospital, no matter how swanky and covered in soft plastic furnishings it is.

And so begins a game of contraction chicken/guess the width of the uterus – which sees many a couple trying to hold off for as long as they can, but secretly scared shitless that they will leave it too late and be left alone with the hot towels and the marigolds.

It's a very good idea at this stage to try to time the contractions, from when they first come on to when they begin to ease off, and then also the space between them. That's two stopwatches worth. This will at least give you a rough guide as to how labour is progressing and as a rule of thumb, you don't need to go to hospital until your partner's contractions last at least 45 seconds and come five to 10 minutes apart.

But if you're in any doubt whatsoever, don't be all British about it and think it best not to bother the midwife; it's absolutely what she's there for and she'll be able to tell an awful lot just by hearing how your partner sounds on the phone. If this is your first baby you'll have no real idea what's coming next so leave the informed guesswork to your seventh, eighth and ninth labours when you will be probably running a sweepstake on when you'll reach the 10cm mark.

Also, if your partner has any semblance of a symptom she is worried about, from the colour of her show, to a headache or worries about the baby's movements – get on the phone and get it checked it out. If the midwife is at all concerned about how you're coping, or even if she just wants to check your partner in person, she will call you in for an assessment. There's a strong chance that you will then be sent home again to wait for things to move along a bit further before going back in. It's frustrating, but unavoidable.

While you are both at home, try to encourage your partner to stay as relaxed and rested as she possibly can, given that every few minutes she is laid low with an ever-increasing pain. She could watch a favourite film, take a warm (but not hot) bath or just try her best to put her feet up in between the contractions. If she feels hungry, eating and drinking something she fancies is a brilliant move to gain some fuel for the heavy, heavy going ahead.

When she's having a contraction, help her to get in whatever position gives her the most relief. Now's also the time to start using any breathing or relaxation techniques you'd learnt at your antenatal classes.

This early stage is also when a TENS (transcutaneous electrical nerve stimulation) machine can be of some use. This little box of tricks sends electrical pulses through your partner's back via pads placed at bra strap and lower back level.

No one really knows how TENS works, but it seems to. It may

stimulate your partner's body to produce endorphins, it may prevent pain signals reaching her brain or it may just be that it's such a bloody palaver to use that it acts as a distraction to what's actually happening.

Endless fiddling with the TENS machine is high on the list of things to keep the expectant father occupied and some men become so attached to them that the machine has to be prised from their hands long after the birth is over. Or at least that's what happened to me.

Time to make a move

As the contractions really start to kick in, you'll decide that it's time to hit the road. Every woman copes with labour pain differently and when it's her time to go in, it's her time to go in.

When you arrive at hospital it would be lovely to say that you will be greeted at the door by the midwife who has coached, cared and caressed your partner for the past nine months, but, especially if you live in a city, the chances are that you won't know her.

Whoever it is though will almost certainly go through the same procedure – they will ask what's happened so far, take a look at your partner's maternity notes and carry out a series of checks on blood pressure, temperature and urine, if there's any of the latter to be had. She will also measure and feel the bump to ascertain which way round your baby is and whether the head is fully engaged in the pelvis. Once that's all done your partner may be asked if she would like an internal examination to find out how dilated she is.

This can be a crushing moment. If your partner has been really suffering contraction-wise and feels like she must be a fair way down the road, only to find out that she is only 1cm–2cm gone, the wind can be knocked out of her. So be prepared to be there for her and tell her how fantastically she is doing.

Now's potentially a good time to get the birth plan out too if you like – double checking with your partner of course that she doesn't want you to put a big red pen through the painkiller-free bit first.

Pain relief

As the contractions become ever more powerful and painful, and your partner moves towards being fully dilated, the pain relief options available to her come into play.

Here's a quick guided tour through what's on offer on the drugs trolley.

Gas and air

Otherwise known as Entonox, this colourless and odourless gas comprises of half oxygen and half nitrous oxide – or laughing gas. The gas enters your partner's bloodstream via a two-way mouthpiece or mask just as a contraction is starting. It has the effect of dampening the pain, relaxing the muscles and making her feel a little light-headed, sometimes, just sometimes even making her laugh. It's definitely worth sneaking a quick slug of it yourself if you find a discreet and opportune moment – but don't have too much for Christ's sake.

Gas and air is most often used at the end of the first stage of labour as contractions intensify in frequency and strength. Some women swear by the stuff, but for others it just isn't strong enough, or the light-headedness or even nausea that it can cause puts them off.

In terms of any effects on the baby, the gas is quickly flushed from the system and there is even evidence to suggest that the high oxygen content is good for the little mite.

Pethidine

Pethidine is a proper painkiller, part of the opiate family and is very similar to morphine. In fact it is morphine, just a synthetic version.

It's mainly administered via injection and is only given during the first stage of labour. There's no doubt pethidine will help your partner relax; it essentially makes the person as high as a kite and gets to work in no time at all. It means business does pethidine.

It doesn't slow down labour either, just dulls the pain significantly, although not totally. Sounds great, I'll have some right away please.

Whoa there, pethidine has its issues. For starters one in three people find opiate drugs such as pethidine unpleasant and the drowsiness, nausea or even bouts of sickness it can bring on are not pleasant.

But pethidine's main drawback is that it crosses the placenta, in other words the baby takes it as well as the mother. The effects this can have range from affecting your baby's breathing and make him drowsy for several days afterwards, to potentially also stifling the baby's rooting and sucking reflexes in the days after birth – making breastfeeding more difficult.

These types of problem seem to be particularly present if your partner's birth progresses more quickly than expected and the baby is born within two hours of the drug being administered.

Meptid and diamorphine – or heroin to you and me – is also often available for labouring women. Both are opiates and have similar advantages and disadvantages to pethidine.

Your partner will not become a heroin fiend as a result of choosing to use diamorphine. I thought that was worth clarifying.

Epidural

The Johnny big bananas of all labour pain relief, an epidural sees painkilling drugs passed into the small of the back via a fine tube.

An anaesthetist administers a local anaesthetic in the lower back and then inserts a hollow needle between the small bones in the spine. The needle then slides into the space between the layers of tissue in your partner's spinal column, handily called the epidural space, and a fine tube is then passed through the needle. Wincing yet? The needle is then removed and the tube taped up your partner's back and over her shoulder. The drug is then injected around the nerves that carry signals from the part of her body that feels the labour pain.

And my word it's become a wildly popular procedure too – official figures show that the numbers of mothers-to-be who have had an epidural has risen in recent years to a whopping 36.5% of all births in the UK [39].

An epidural can be given at any point in labour, but the majority of women go for this option when their contractions are getting pretty fierce as the cervix moves towards its full dilation.

There's one big, shining benefit of the epidural route – it more often than not provides excellent pain relief during labour. The mind remains perfectly clear unlike via the pethidine route and while your partner will be aware of the contractions she's having, if the epidural is working correctly, she will feel no pain. That's quite a draw.

It's not without its problems and risks though – and there are quite a few to consider:

> Firstly, the buttock clenching procedure itself takes about 20 minutes itself and another 20 minutes for the anaesthetic to kick in – which may not happen first time of asking.

> Your baby's heartbeat and your partner's blood pressure will be monitored continuously for at least 30 minutes when she's first given an epidural, and after each top-up of the anaesthetic if it's needed. There's also a higher risk of the labour needing to be speeded up using a hormone drip once an epidural has been given.

> Not being in full control of the nether regions can also mean that the pushing stage of the delivery may last longer with an epidural.

> Itching, fever or the shivers can occur and your partner may also need a catheter to empty her bladder.

> There's a higher chance of your baby needing to be born with the aid of ventouse or forceps, which may be because epidurals make it difficult for your baby to move into the best position for him to be born.

> There's also a very small risk of the procedure leading to nerve damage. Although this rarely happens, the risk is about one in 1,000 for temporary damage and one in 13,000 for permanent problems.

The wider debate about the benefits of drug-free births is a thorny and complex one, with one of the UK's most prominent midwives recently suggesting that the increase in pain relief during labour undermines the mother's bond with her child [40].

All I'll say is that if men delivered the babies, we would be asking for all of the above in giant pill form – to be applied suppositorily at five-minute intervals.

Transition

Maybe it's because it sounds a bit like intermission, but whenever anyone mentioned the transition phase of pregnancy I conjured up images of a small oasis of calm in which people come into the room selling choc-ices and you are invited to nip to the loo if you like, or go and put some more change in the parking meter. I got that very wrong.

The transition phase is for many women the most difficult part of the entire labour; the point where even the steeliest of resolves to avoid pain relief are tested to the maximum. This is the point when the cervix moves from around 8cm to the full 10cm dilation, and the second, pushing stage of the pregnancy can begin.

It's often said that contractions become less frequent at this point, but that's only really because they become so long and strong that they seem to merge into one. It's also common for your partner's waters to break as this stage begins and she may also get an urge to do a poo, as this is the time when the baby's head touches the rectum. That urge may well turn into a reality too, although your partner may or may not be aware of the comings and goings down there. If it does happen do your best to play the whole thing down – it's as natural as having the baby itself and your partner shouldn't feel embarrassed for a single second.

Getting her through it

Transition is a tough, tough time and it can often be arrived at after many hours of energy and spirit sapping early labour too. Helping your partner through this often dark period is one of the most important jobs you'll ever do. That help can come in many ways: physically helping her to find the best position, comforting her if she feels shaky or shivery, encouraging her to release the guttural, almost cattle-like noises she is making, or ensuring her pain relief choices happen – no matter how much they might differ from the birth plan.

It might just be though that you need to bear the brunt of some pretty fruity and forceful outbursts from the love of your life. Don't be surprised if you are showered with more than the odd volley of obscenities as each contraction takes hold – there's even scientific evidence that swearing does actually alleviate pain [41], so she has every excuse, not that she needed one of course.

Whatever it takes, getting to the next stage is the name of the game, because at the end of that, you are going to see your baby for the very first time.

Almost there

The cervix is fully open and your partner is ready – or as ready as she'll ever be – to push her baby out into the world.

If she's lucky she may well have experienced a spell without any contractions in between transition and this, the second stage of pregnancy, called in some quarters the rest-and-be-thankful phase. If that little spell of calm didn't exist you'd imagine the childbirth marketing board would invent it to give labouring mothers the tiniest of life rafts to cling to.

Although there are different approaches to pushing, the one that is overwhelmingly favoured by UK midwives is that women push when they get the strong urge to do so and rest when they don't – the other largely discredited method being that they push throughout once they have reached full dilation.

With every push and contraction – which at this stage are around 60–90 seconds long and come at two to four minute intervals – the baby will move through the pelvis a little, but as the urge dies away he'll probably slip back a bit again too – fear not though progress will be made, albeit slowly.

Gone are the days when women dutifully lay flat on the bed, legs up so the doctor didn't have to strain his neck to see what was going on and attempted to essentially push against gravity. Out of bed positions are becoming more and more popular and it's not hard to see why – squatting for instance opens the pelvic area by an additional 10%. Birth stools and balls as well as water pools are all options to be considered and if it's where your partner wants to go, it's your job to help make it happen.

Whichever position does it for your partner, the art of pushing effectively these days is characterised by her not holding her breath and turning purple, but rather going with the contractions and the urge, burying her chin into her chest, letting out a deep growl and pushing through her bottom as if she were having a nice poo – which again, she may well do.

Once the baby's head is way down the pelvis and your partner can feel the burning sensation that characterises crowning – when the baby's head starts to stretch the opening to the vagina – you really are getting close.

Assisted deliveries

But things don't always go smoothly, in fact one in eight UK births are assisted using instruments. There are several reasons why an assisted birth might be recommended. Your baby might be getting distressed as he is being pushed down the birth canal, or he may not be budging much at all, or your partner simply might have zero energy left to push with. So what high tech tools has modern medicine developed to help in this delicate procedure then?

A plunger and some giant medieval tongs.

The plunger is of course the ventouse; a cup with a pulling handle attached to it, which is linked to a small vacuum pump. Sophisticated, it's not.

The cup fits on top, and the back of your baby's head is held firm (ishly) by the vacuum and the cup is then pulled on during the next contraction. This will be tried around three times to see if the little one can be convinced to make an appearance.

Be warned: babies born using the ventouse sometimes come out with cone-shaped heads or looking like they are wearing some sort of Olympic cycling helmet. This effect of the suction almost always wears off after a few days.

Despite being a pretty basic way of helping a delicate little baby along its way, the ventouse is positively feather-like compared with the other instrument available – forceps. These satanic salad servers come in two interlocked parts, and have curved ends to cradle your baby's head.

Your doctor will need to make a cut to the back of your partner's vagina, called an episiotomy, so the forceps can be inserted to put round the sides of your baby's head. Once they are in place, the doctor will gently pull during a contraction to try to lever the baby out of his hidey hole.

Although forceps have a higher success rate than ventouse, your partner is also more likely to sustain some damage with their use. As it is much more painful, there is also a higher chance of her needing an anaesthetic to be able to cope with the use of forceps.

Most forceps births are straightforward, although your partner may experience some soreness and bruising afterwards. Your baby may be slightly bruised too and conditions such as torticollis (wry neck), which result from damage to the neck muscles during the procedure, should be looked out for in the weeks after birth.

If after three attempts with the forceps your baby is still refusing to move it's almost certainly time to stop tugging and think about a caesarean section.

A caesarean section (c-section) involves making an incision into the woman's abdomen and uterus to manually remove the baby. Most c-sections are performed under epidural rather than general anaesthesia, and if this is decided on, you will be able to stay with your partner throughout. A screen is usually put up while it takes place so you and your partner don't have to witness what's going on – many men can't resist a peek though and some regret it given what they then see.

While a c-section is a serious medical procedure, it can be over remarkably quickly and before you know where you are, after hours and hours of labour you can suddenly be holding your new baby.

Delivering the placenta and the stitch-up job can take half an hour, so you become the caregiver for the baby there and then. As you'd expect after having major surgery, your partner will be pretty immobile and in considerable pain for a good while afterwards, meaning your role once you get home becomes even more crucial too.

The number of caesareans is on the increase, in 2007/8 almost 25% of all births happened that way, either by women choosing to go that route or ending up having to. Natural childbirth campaigners, such as the NCT have expressed concerns over the trend [42].

It's a baby

If your partner is fortunate enough to avoid having an assisted birth in any of its forms, the midwife will tell her that she can see the baby's head and that he is no longer slipping back between each contraction. After a pause from pushing on the next contraction or two, to help ensure that the baby is born nice and gently, and to help avoid any tears or the need for a last-minute episiotomy, the final pushes will begin.

As the majority of babies finally emerge, they do so with their chin down on their chest. Once the head is fully out one shoulder is delivered, swiftly followed by the other one and the rest of the body slides out at quite a pace.

However your baby is delivered, whatever your partner has to go through to help your little one make the final few inches towards life on the outside, there will come a moment when you both get to see your baby boy or girl for the very first time in the flesh. After hours or even days of unprecedented effort your truly amazing partner has achieved something so extraordinary that you'll never quite see her in the same way ever again – she's moved from woman to superwoman.

Then, covered in blood, cream cheese and amniotic fluid, your baby will be handed to your partner and neither of you will have seen anything so amazingly beautiful in your entire lives.

You my friend, are a father.

Congratulations.

Tying up loose ends

Immediately after your baby is born, if all is well with both mother and child, skin-to-skin contact will be established between the two without delay to start the bonding process. There's also plenty of evidence to suggest that you should get your shirt off and get close to your little one too at some point, as well as fixing his gaze with yours – both of which are thought to help form a lasting bond between you and your new child.

One job that needs to be done before you do that is the cutting of the umbilical cord. The midwife will clamp it in two places and if you wish you can do the honours in what has become a well-practiced symbolic gesture of the establishing of true independence. In reality it's like cutting a very tough and gristly German sausage.

Before you can start to really get to know the new arrival and your partner can begin the process of establishing breastfeeding if that's the way you intend to go, there are a few quick tests and measurements that need to be taken.

The baby's airways will be cleared of any mucus and after the weight is recorded, the Apgar score will be taken. This is a simple method to quickly assess the health of newborn children immediately after childbirth by measuring Appearance, Pulse, Grimace, Activity and Respiration. This test is done twice at approximately one and five minutes after birth.

Afterbirth afterthought

While all the loveliness of meeting, bonding and even feeding the newborn little bundle is going on, the third stage of pregnancy, the process of delivering the placenta is already underway. Contractions begin again, although thankfully weaker this time, with the aim of making the placenta gradually come away from the wall of the womb. A lot of hospitals give the new Mum an injection to speed up this process.

It's hard not to feel that this is a pain in the arse – the job has been done and all your partner wants to do is cuddle her new baby. Luckily on most occasions this is a relatively straightforward procedure with the strange bagpipe-like sack of membranes which has kept your child alive just dropping out without much fuss.

In Mali, it's thought that the placenta can affect the baby's mood and it's washed, dried and placed in a basket to be buried by the father. In Cambodia, it's carefully wrapped in a banana leaf, placed beside the newborn for three days and then buried. In South America and Korea, it's ceremonially burned after birth to neutralise it. We tend to put it straight in the bin providing we've not been suckered into turning it into a pâté by Hugh Fearnley-Whittingstall.

Occasionally, getting the placenta out can be much more complicated because leaving even tiny fragments of it inside the uterus can lead to heavy bleeding. When all other avenues have been explored and it hasn't come out, an operation will be required to remove it – meaning that even if a woman has avoided having an epidural to deliver her baby, she may be forced to have one to allow her doctor to remove the placenta manually. As well as being painful and stressful for your partner, this means that you are Charles in charge when it comes to your baby's first hour or so on the planet.

And breathe

Your first experience of childbirth will never leave you. Shocking or sentimental, traumatic or transformational – the memories of the moment you became a father and what your partner went through to make that happen will live as long as you do.

No matter what friends who've been there tell you ahead of the event, no matter what you see on the television or at the movies and no matter what you read, yes even in books like this one, nothing even gets close to how you will feel.

As you leave the hospital and begin to call or text friends and relatives with the big news you will be physically drained, emotionally spent and probably not smelling too great either, but chances are you'll be as happy, as genuinely, undoubtedly happy as you've ever been.

Cherish every moment of this day and the days that follow it as you burst with pride for your new family – it really is life at its very best.

Stories from the frontline

The birth story is, quite rightly, the preserve of the mother.

In the weeks and months after your child is born you will hear it told and retold, mainly to other women, all of whom listen intently. Those who have recently given birth themselves will wait for a suitable moment to cut in with their own story and the ones yet to experience childbirth will sit dead still, the colour draining from their cheeks, as they wonder whether they could cope.

But just this once, just because we can, let's hear what it was like for the fathers. Alright, so we've not had the unspeakable pain, the needles in our spine or the stitches in our unmentionables, but we were there, we were there.

Chris, 34, father of one *We arrived at the hospital at about 8am. Anouk was born at 8.47am. So we held on at home with those contractions a fair while!*

They did say come in at the last possible moment. My wife actually collapsed in the reception – apparently the receptionists hate women having babies in the reception area, so my wife was quickly ushered to her feet and up we went to the birthing room.

I'm an old hippie, so remember hoping that my wife would get in the bath for a water birth and as it turned out she actually was up for it, but couldn't get over to the bath. Anouk was on the way, born on the floor of the birthing room. I remember being fascinated at the way the head turns and the shoulders squash up to get out... and being slightly amused when the midwife asked my wife if she wanted a mirror (to see what was going on – she didn't – obviously).

Colin, 33, father of one: *After I got 'the call' at work to say Susanne's waters had broken I responded in time-honoured fashion and prepared to race home there and then, only to be told to stop being a numpty and come home after work... this was going to take a while.*

And it did.

That evening we went for a long walk and a curry and at around midnight the contractions really started to kick in. We phoned the hospital and they told us to come in. Susanne was examined and told she was only 1cm dilated and we went home again, arriving at about 6am.

At about 5pm that evening the contractions were getting fast and quite strong and at sevenish I called the hospital back and was told they were full. Full, like an NCP car park.

The suggestion we were given was to go to another hospital nearby – one which we had heard from friends with firsthand experience was horrific. So we waited as long as we dared and I called back at about 10pm hoping against hope that it would be open – and it was.

We raced in, expecting to be near the big moment, but no, Susanne was still only 1cm. But at least we were in the bloody place now and nothing was going to shift us.

Susanne took some pethidine and we managed to get four hours much needed rest, my big fear was that when things did eventually get moving she would be completely and totally spent, having been in labour for almost two days already. So its 4am now, the pethidine has all but worn off and its time for another examination. 4cm.

Four hours later – 6cm. The following examination two hours after that, still 6cm.

That was when things suddenly got very clinical. We were taken to theatre where Susanne was put on a monitor and given a hormone drip to increase the contractions. Serious pain at this point – and it later turned out Isabella was 'back to back' – so Susanne decided she wanted an epidural.

As the anaesthetist was attempting to find the right spot in her back for the injection the baby's heart rate kept on plummeting and for the first time I began to contemplate something going seriously wrong.

Then Susanne let out an almighty scream and there was the head! Bin the epidural and push, push, push. More than 90 minutes later after trying stirrups and birthing chairs, the midwife called the doctor with the ventouse.

Luckily, before she could get that far, Isabella popped out aided with a few snips from the massive scissors.

A huge, huge effort from my wife and one I will never forget or stop admiring her for.

Donald, 34, father of two: *Quite near the end of the pregnancy my wife had woken up screaming in pain during the middle of the night and I immediately thought this is it... but when I realised it was a merely a bit of cramp I soon fell fast asleep, after performing the obligatory 'leg in the air rub the calf' footballer's treatment of course.*

I won't call it crying wolf, but when my wife woke me again 10 minutes before my alarm was due to sound for work and said her waters had broken I'll admit it took me a while for things to register, but once the penny had dropped I sprung to life. Our first visit to the hospital – like many on their big day – was in vain and we were sent home with the advice that she should be going into the early stages of labour by the close of play that night.

When she did go into labour at about 3pm that afternoon my parents, who had been notified early, decided they would show up unannounced... bad idea. By this point the contractions had started and the doorbell went. We were mystified as to who it could be but a simple peak out the window alerted us to it being my parents. My Japanese wife, who never ever shouts, screamed, 'Get them out of here, they are not coming in.'

I ushered my parents away before they even caught sight of my wife but left them with the news that she may be going into labour (resulting in a machine gun-like response by way of text messages over the hours that followed).

I got back to my wife who was clearly in pain and (forgetting all I had been told and shown in my NCT classes) I tried to massage her back during contractions instead of between – an error of quite enormous proportions. 'Get your fucking hands off me!' Wow! My wife who never shouts and certainly never swears suddenly does both – very well!'

I took that as my cue to call the hospital and spoke to a midwife, who was surprisingly unhelpful. She said she could hear by the sound of my wife in the background that she is clearly not ready and we would only be sent home – now that is talent bordering on the supernatural. She said I can't tell you not to come, but I believe you will be wasting your time. Bugger her I thought, rush hour is on its way and my wife's newly discovered expletive vocabulary would surely expand rapidly should we get stuck in traffic, so we left at once.

At the hospital we were quickly shown to a room and then left completely on our own for about 40 minutes. My wife was in such excruciating pain that I slightly lost it and told the desk of doctors, nurses and midwives to stop chatting among themselves and get someone in to look at my wife... please. This seemed to do the trick and a midwife followed me back very casually. She was less casual when she took one look at the business end of my wife and shouted 'Don't push, you're 10cm dilated and I can see the head!'.

From then on we had what felt like hundreds of midwives crowded around the water birth pool. I was made chief fisherman in case unusual pieces of... well anything should appear in the water. At one point when the baby's head had nearly come out and my wife's contractions stopped she promptly fell fast asleep. We all started shouting at her and she awoke startled like she'd been sleeping for hours. After an initial look of sheer bewilderment she remembered where she was and went straight back to the push and grind... I was so impressed and still am.

When Emily was born – I cut the cord and she was passed to me. She opened her eyes and two blue marbles looked up at me... it was amazing... the world stopped.

It wasn't quite over for the wife though, the senior midwife asked if a student doctor could deliver the placenta, which she did, only for it to fire out and explode in the student's face. Her hair was covered, her glasses were red, and her chin was dripping. We never did find out whether this young fresh-faced girl did pursue a medical career or finish her course or even make it to the shower.

Going home to an empty house that night was very strange. I was so excited I wanted to celebrate and wake the world. Unfortunately it was now about 1am on a school night and I had to make do with a couple of cold beers on my own, while mulling over the events of the day. This was not out of the ordinary, kids are born all over the world all the time but nevertheless 'new life' was amazing!

Jim, 34, father of one: *We had a 26-hour labour all in. For the first 20 hours I was pretty relaxed, and thought we were all doing well. I was in control and going to boss the situation.*

The next three hours were really long, draining and increasingly worrying. It began to get a little messy. The dried apricots failed to re-energise anyone and I had forgotten the sandwiches in the car. I could not do the mantra anywhere near as good as the midwife. Gooood, Gooood, Very Gooooooooooood, my timing was not up to scratch and I had no idea she was coordinating her Goods with breathing and pushing. I took some stick for that!

The next two hours were increasingly alarming and I began to think these people did not know what they were doing, we could see Paul's little head, but they couldn't get him out. My partner's face was red and full of burst blood vessels.

The last hour consisted of an emotional schizophrenia, the like of which I've never experienced before – horrified/serene/angry/ grateful/scared/proud and back to the beginning again. I had no idea, no control, so I just held my Anne all the time, taking the squeezes, the pinches but thankfully no punches.

She was incredible. The most amazing woman – incredible to think all Mums have been through this. I look at mothers in a different light now.

On arrival Paul looked like a shrunken scraggy old man, and a lot like my nan.

Levi, 36, father of two: *It's not quick like on the telly with rushing and hot towels and then birth. Labour was long and boring, and watching your wife in regular, gut-wrenching pain is not fun at all.*

You're also excited, but you want this bit over. Like when you have to finish something truly horrible on your plate before getting a big bowl of crème caramel. I only felt useful at the end, when my wife was being urged to really push, and I held her hand and counted to 10 with her and urged her on. A bit like a boxing coach in the corner but without pouring cold water on her genitals.

Our child was forceps-delivered. I thought the doctor was pulling my wife off the bed at one point. Horrendous, and the baby was born with red marks on her jaw when the clamps were fitted.

We had agreed that I only had one job and that was to tell my wife if we'd had a boy or a girl. The moment was so shocking that I could only splutter in wonder 'It's a baby', much to the midwives' mirth.

I cut the cord, but only because I was asked if I wanted to and not because I felt like I was giving life to this bundle – I didn't, my wife did that bit. People who think cutting the cord is really meaningful and symbolic are dreaming.

You wait all day in an unpleasant, hot, pretty sterile, not particularly chilled-out environment. You're worried and everything takes ages. You've waited nine months for this day. Nine months is an unexpectedly long time. You know it's coming, that's why we're all here, isn't it? Yet, I was STILL gobsmacked when a baby came into the room. An extra person was magicked in there. An awesome feeling.

I drove home at great speed, exhilarated and listening to Mozart at full blast in the middle of the night. I thought about my Dad too, and felt very happy.

Nick, 35, father of two: *We had a planned c-section. It was incredibly weird going out for dinner the night before knowing that we were going to have a baby the next morning. Sleep was at a premium that night too.*

The taxi driver knew and wished us luck! The theatre was strange – a place of work for the staff in there, something inevitable and predictable for everyone except us.

Then he came out – he looked exactly like my Dad – my wife had given birth to my Dad. ... it was... surreal and amazing.

Peter, 33, father of one:
Many things stand out from the birth for me, but there were a few key moments. First of all it was the only day of the year it snowed and a 20-minute journey took about an hour and a quarter – including a bit of skidding on icy roundabouts and 10mph on the dual carriageway in blizzard conditions. Despite really close

and hard contractions my darling wife still felt compos mentis enough to criticise my driving – but at least it took her mind off the impending pushing.

When we finally got to the hospital as always I was told I'd parked in the wrong spot and was made to find another despite the contractions coming long and hard. Once we were inside my wife was off her face on the gas and air. So much so, she actually couldn't remember how to push when the moment came. However, the mild threat that a doctor may have to be brought in to examine her when there was a 15-minute lull got things moving very sharpish. I remember that just like in the sitcoms you can actually hear the occasional primal scream from elsewhere in the unit. It's odd to admit but even when you get near to the very end it always takes 10 times as long as you think. A minute seems like an hour.

The only scary moment was when Sam came into the world the midwife pressed the emergency button, but that was just to get another midwife to help her cut the umbilical cord. For a split second I thought there were massive problems, but everything was ok.

In contrast the most emotional moment of the lot was telling my wife that we'd had a boy. Actually seeing him brought tears to my eyes and my voice went all wobbly. I didn't feel instant love – I was in awe of the little fella; how he had all these toes and fingers and how he knew he should breath. Just incredible.

And the most surreal experience was about 30 minutes after Sam was born. The midwife told us Alex had a tear that needed stitches. A couple of minutes later a small doctor came in asked her to open her legs before he put them in stirrups. 'Pretend I'm not here' he said, before strapping a kind of pot-holing light to his forehead, turning it on and proceeding to insert the stitches.

As we attempted to talk softly and gaze lovingly at each other and our new son the thread was lifted high into the air time and again as this tiny little doctor with a miner's lamp on stitched my wife's nether regions.

Stuart, 37, father of two: *After an unsuccessful induction attempt at the doctor's we were told to ring the hospital a few days later and as we were almost two weeks overdue at this point we were up bright and early ready to go.*

After initially being told there were no beds, we called back again and got the go-ahead to come in, so picked up our bags and travelled in style to the hospital on the bus. After being induced a second time we were told that it could take a while and despite going for a walk to get things moving so it proved.

It wasn't until 8 or 9 at night when the contractions started to kick in by which time my partner was on the antenatal ward, meaning I had to leave, which was a nightmare knowing that she had a night of pain ahead of her, but they insisted and kicked me out.

After a restless night's sleep at home with the phone on my pillow I made my way back to the hospital as soon as I was allowed in to find my partner in even more pain and having had no sleep at all. The fact that she had to go through that night on her own was a scandal.

By 3 o'clock that afternoon we were in full flow with the birthing plan thrown out of the window and the epidural administered. By 10 that night our daughter still refused to enter the world and there was talk of an emergency caesarean which would have suited me fine because by this point my better half looked totally shattered after 24 hours of labour.

Luckily though she is made of stern stuff and had a bit more fight to push, and with a little help from a scalpel Lily was born at 1.13am.

A few hours of getting to know my new little girl were magical before I was kicked out again to do the ring round, float home and then float back again first thing.

Suki, 34, father of two: *The first time around we went into hospital two or three days on the trot after minor contractions* had started, only to be told baby wasn't ready each time. Once the waters had partly broken, we went back and then had to start on what turned out to be a 20+ hour process of induction, which ended, as a lot of them do I believe, in a forceps delivery.

I was totally exhausted so I can't even begin to imagine how my wife felt. The arrival of the baby was simply the best feeling ever; the Mum carries it for nine long months and to be able to finally hold this tiny little being yourself is fantastic.

Tom, 34, father of two: *I remember my back killing me during the labour and as my wife had had an epidural by then I popped on a redundant TENS machine – queue funny looks from midwives of course.*

I mainly juggled monitoring the monitor with keeping the music fresh. And once we got down to crunch time, I even managed to use the rose petal spray, which was both ineffective and camp all at once.

We were far more casual the second time around. Arrived nicely dilated thanks to my magnificent wife, worked through the following hours superbly and because Jane seemed so in control I could really focus on the music.

Both arrived to Norah Jones, God bless that woman.

Oli, 35, father of one: *The birth was horrible to be honest.*

Firstly if you like to be in control, then this is the one moment when you're not, you mostly hang around, generally on the fringes of what is going on.

I hate hospitals anyway and don't like needles, so when they did the epidural, I went out the room. I was very emotional, particularly as we had an emergency Caesarean.

Both A and J were in a lot of distress, so after about four hours they rushed us in to do the caesarean.

Seeing someone you love in immense pain and distress, particularly when you can't do anything is horrible. When people say, it's a wonderful experience, I think that's bollocks, in my mind get it over and done with ASAP.

David, 34, father of one: *After 10 days of curries, pineapple and anatomically awkward, but surprisingly sexy sex we had to face the truth – we were going to be induced.*

Arriving at hospital I was utterly amazed just how calm my wife was. To me this was like a horror film – voluntarily checking yourself into somewhere in the absolute knowledge that unbearable pain was the unavoidable conclusion.

But she was cool. She's been happier obviously, but so strong was the desire to finally see the baby that had been inside her for what seemed like three and a half years, that she was virtually guiding the midwife in like an air traffic controller when the time came to apply the gel.

Despite what we had read, contractions didn't begin there and then with a fearful and thunderous crash.

In fact, nothing happened, so we went for a walk and even decided to go for some pasta at a place near the hospital to boost our energy levels for the night ahead.

About three hours later my wife started to feel back aches and mild stomach cramps which got worse pretty quickly – and we knew things were starting.

By the time Sarah got into bed on the pre maternity ward she was in a fair bit of pain but still pretty calm. When the nurse came round and we told her we thought labour was starting she came out with the classic line that it couldn't be labour because my wife looked too happy and if it was labour she'd know about it.

Wrong.

The time was gone 11pm and it was kicking out time on the ward for men, including me and I was ushered out – leaving Sarah in increasing pain. After half an hour pacing outside the hospital I knew I had to go back in and tailgated someone through the doors. When I got to Sarah's bed she was out like a light and the midwife, surprised to see me back, told me that she had been given pethodine after asking for painkilling help.

Even more worried that things would soon be kicking off I pleaded to stay but was told to leave the ward, go home and get some sleep – as soon as anything was looking like happening I'd be called, but they didn't think anything would be happening for hours.

Wrong again.

Just as I walked in the front door of our house after a half hour drive my mobile rang and I was told my wife was about to start pushing and that I needed to rush back.

I raced back and was just in time for the start of the pushing phase – she had gone through full dilation on her own.

The pushing stage was thankfully very quick and almost straightforward and an hour and a half after it had started we had a beautiful baby boy.

And we thought that was that. But it wasn't. The bloody placenta refused to come out, despite the midwife pawing at it like James Herriot. A full two litres of blood later and the doctor was finally called. She took one look and whisked my poor wife off to theatre to have an epidural so they could get the placenta out with impunity. Resisting an epidural for the baby but being forced to have one for the placenta felt like a real kick in the teeth for my wife, but soon enough the trauma began to fade for her.

It goes without saying though that we will be giving that hospital a miss should we be lucky enough to have a next time.

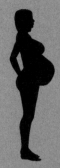

MONTH 9.5

Being overdue

As we've seen, the due date of your baby is a rough estimate at best and a load of old cobblers at worst. But even with that knowledge lodged in your partner's brain, the very second the given date comes and goes you are officially overdue. It's a blunt word for a pretty blunt time and one which unites womankind in frustration, uncomfortableness and not a little irritation.

Once your partner reaches her 41st week she will be checked out by an obstetrician to see if the aforementioned dodgy due date really is dodgy. The position of the baby will be checked as well as its size and there may even be an internal examination carried out to see whether the cervix feels soft and ready for labour or hard and ready for a fight.

You may also be offered a sweep – a word which will take on a whole new meaning to you in the coming days. It refers to the procedure of sweeping the membranes, which while sounding like a grunge band from Devon, is actually a medical procedure and a pretty unsophisticated one at that. It involves the midwife or doctor sweeping a finger around the cervix during an internal examination to try to separate the membranes around the baby from the cervix itself. This in turn releases hormones which could kick-start labour. It won't come as a shock to anyone to discover that having a sweep can be somewhat uncomfortable or even downright painful – but it does increase the likelihood that labour will start within 48 hours and poses no risk of infection whatsoever.

As a manual introduction to induction it's worth a go, because the medical alternatives that come into view as time ticks on don't take many prisoners.

A helping hand

Nobody wants to be induced.

Apocryphal stories abound of going from nought to 10cm dilation in 90 seconds and contractions so strong that they cause structural damage to the hospital.

So why don't we all just wait until the little 'un is good and ready?

The reason overdue mothers-to-be make obstetricians very nervous indeed is because the risk of the placenta beginning to fail in its task of keeping the baby alive increases ever so slightly as the pregnancy goes past full term. The risk of stillbirth in the UK is around one per 3,000 pregnancies at 39 weeks, four per 3,000 at 42 weeks and eight per 3,000 at 43 weeks. It's those figures that are the driving force behind the fact that in England something like one in every five women is induced.

Once the membrane sweep has been tried and is unsuccessful, a range of induction options will be offered to your partner. She by this time will not only be climbing the walls wanting to get her enormous child out of her body but also swearing on all that is holy – the next person to ask if there's any news will be attacked with a fully charged TENS machine.

The midwife or doctor may also arrive at something called the Bishop's score, which is a scoring system to predict if an induction is required and/or would be successful. Based on five elements assessed during an internal examination, a grade from 0 to 13 is given. A score above 9 means labour will still most likely start spontaneously, anything beneath 6 and an induction is probably needed.

Five and the bonus ball and you could pay your mortgage off.

The 'natural' way

It's a measure of just how pissed off overdue women get at not being able to get shot of their stowaway that over the years that they have been prepared to try so many bizarre and more often than not bollocks ways of starting off labour. Here are just the merest handful.

Sex

Now, let me see, I wonder who could have come up with this? So determined was the man who cooked up this one that he even took the time to invent three separate ways in which it works.

Firstly, orgasm helps to stimulate the womb into action (a little presumptuous given how logistically difficult the act of sex is at this stage, never mind good sex). Secondly, semen helps to ripen or soften the neck of the womb (the guidance is unclear whether this should be applied directly or taken orally). And thirdly, the jiggy-jiggy nature of sex itself can kick things off.

You've got to admire him for his thoroughness, but it's almost certainly a load of old twaddle.

Castor oil

Taking castor oil to bring on labour is an ancient trick that is thought to get the uterus going by serving up a bad case of diarrhoea, with a side order of nausea.

While a few small studies have shown this to be somewhat effective, the dehydration that can be caused at such a critical time marks this method of induction down as only slightly less mad than hanging your partner out of the window by her ankles until things get a move on.

Eating pineapple

The enzyme bromelain, which is found in fresh pineapples (canned or juiced varieties lose it) is thought in some quarters to help soften the cervix.

Given the tiny amount of the enzyme in each pineapple your partner will need to eat a lorry load, by which time she will such a case of the shits that she will no longer be aware she is still alive, never mind still pregnant.

Eating curry

Almost certainly another poo-related method.

Homoeopathy

Who knows whether the root of the shoot of the root of the lesser nettle buckweed shrub, or whatever is the recommended potion, actually does anything, but one thing is for sure: when a homoeopathist puts a bottle of tiny, tiny tablets into an overdue woman's hand and says under absolutely no circumstances should she take any more than one of those tablets, you can be assured of a couple of things:

> ❭ The woman will believe that these tablets hold the answer to her prayers.

> ❭ She will take five of them.

What doesn't help is when her husband then tells her that they taste like tic-tacs and are almost certainly a placebo. Take it from me, not a good move.

The last resort

The final and almost foolproof way of bringing on labour is for the expectant father to drink two bottles of red wine very quickly. He is almost guaranteed to be required to drive to the hospital within the hour, but will end up being forced to drunkenly beg taxi firms to ignore their 'no amniotic fluid on the leather policy' and take them in.

The medical way

If your partner has made love to a pineapple while munching on a castor oil-drenched onion bhaji and there's still no movement as she approaches the 42nd week mark, the medical induction options come into play.

Prostaglandin

Prostaglandin is a hormone-like substance, which helps stimulate uterine contractions and can be administered via a gel, pessary or tablet into the vagina. The drug tends to kick in over the course of a few hours, although a second dose can sometimes be needed.

There's a very small risk that, as with Syntocinon below, the uterus may become over-stimulated or hyper-stimulated, which can reduce the amount of oxygen getting to your baby – if this happens drugs are given to slow things down.

Syntocinon

Syntocinon, a synthetic form of the hormone oxytocin is only given if prostaglandin has failed to do its thing. Your partner would be given this via an intravenous drip, meaning it goes straight into the bloodstream. Syntocinon is a powerful drug and can cause strong contractions that could put the baby under stress, meaning continuous monitoring is necessary. Women who are given Syntocinon often choose to have an epidural as contractions brought on via this route can be more painful than natural ones. You may also be offered a caesarean before choosing to try Syntocinon.

Artificially rupturing the membranes

This is a scary sounding method of breaking the waters that is fast becoming a thing of the past or a last resort if for some reason prostaglandin can't be given.

A midwife or doctor makes a small tear in the membranes around the baby using either a probe with a hook on the end, or a glove with a needle-like prick at the end of one of the fingers.

The words Jesus and wept spring to mind.

Coping

With the prospect of induction looming larger every day that baby chooses to stay put, it's no wonder that the post-40-week phase of a pregnancy can be among the most trying of the whole thing for your partner. Your job is to keep her as calm and as occupied as possible. Sitting in the house and thinking about nothing else is a recipe for a serious case of cabin fever.

Despite the dubious scientific evidence for all the old wives' tales remedies, what they all have going for them is that they give you both something relatively positive and proactive to talk, try and obsess about – although if you are seriously considering the castor oil route it's time to go and see the midwife again!

Remember, 80% of all births don't require induction and if you fall in the remaining 20%, you'll both find a way to get through it, because you are very nearly parents and that's what parents do.

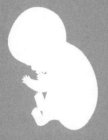

EPILOGUE
Holding a baby

You, your baby and superwoman

Once the sheer drama of childbirth has passed and you have called and texted almost every human being you've ever met, you'll regretfully say goodbye to your new little family and almost certainly drive home, shattered but as happy as you've ever been.

There's something incredibly special about travelling to hospital to visit the two most important people in your life – full of pride, full of love and in awe of what your partner went through. This short little spell before they come home is one of those intensely personal and joyful times in your life that you'll never forget.

Of course for your partner the next few weeks or even months is a period of recovery. In the immediate aftermath there could be tears to be shed, stitches to heal, heavy postnatal bleeding to stem and stretch marks to come to terms with. She could feel elated, delighted, overwhelmed or depressed; childbirth is a huge event and everyone deals with the fall-out in different ways. If she had a caesarean, walking, standing or even just sitting up could be real problems, and your help and support will be vital.

On the plus side, their job done, the hormonal hordes quickly start to slink away meaning the unholy trinity of heartburn, piles and constipation are relieved pretty quickly.

Going home

Postnatal care in the nation's hospitals varies wildly. Some women receive attention, advice and support that genuinely helps them in the testing days and weeks to come. For others the post-delivery ward is a place to escape from as soon as possible. A noisy, impersonal hell hole that stuffs in new Mums and their babies like brooding battery hens.

Either way, after anything from 24 hours to a handful of days (or a week or more in complicated cases) the time to take your baby and its Mum home will come.

After the tentative drive back there will come a moment when you both sit down in the familiar surroundings of the place where you live and the penny will drop – you are parents, you have an utterly dependent little baby and it's down to the pair of you to provide for him and protect him. Bloody hell.

The hard yards

Now isn't the time or the place to go into detail about what the initial weeks and months with your first born baby are like. That would be a whole different book that you would be frankly too utterly shagged out to read anyway.

Of course every couple's experience is different, but it's safe to say that your lack of sleep will soon become something that your tired, tired mind obsesses about – you know it's coming, but you can't prepare for it. Think of it as a rite of parenting passage, something every new Mum and Dad (no matter what they tell you about their 20-second-old baby already sleeping through the night) have to go through before they can really look at other parents, including their own, in the eye and say, we were there!

The other area that seems to cause an inordinate amount of discomfort, anguish and often real pain is breastfeeding. For something so natural, breastfeeding has the ability to drive many new parents to the edge in the very early stages of parenthood, just when they are at their most nervous and vulnerable. There's no shortage of advice, in fact that's often part of the problem with hospital staff promoting one technique, health visitors another and friends and relatives chipping in too.

Sore, cracked or even bleeding nipples as the little one tries unsuccessfully to latch on are sadly quite common and all the while the hungry baby lets its frustration show in the only way he knows how.

Of course breastfeeding can just click the first time of asking, but if it doesn't and it starts to become a struggle it can seriously colour the first few days at home. With the list of known benefits derived from breast milk seemingly growing by the week the pressure to persevere and stick at it can be immense. Many women who have problems eventually move on to the bottle as the painful and worrying days tick by and if that happens your support, reassurance and understanding are crucial.

The march of time

Once the first few difficult weeks have been negotiated you'll no doubt attempt to get into some sort of routine. That's a big ask for a little baby and you may well find yourself up at 4am for the 10th night on the trot wondering what you and your partner are doing wrong. The answer will almost certainly be absolutely nothing.

Despite how those long, long nights might feel at the time, the truth is before you have had time to realise what's going on, your baby will be sitting up, standing up and running off – no matter how hard you find the beginning, the initial few weeks and months of your first baby's life will slip through your fingers at an incredible rate.

Savouring anything when you've not slept properly for days or even weeks is incredibly hard, but that's what you need to do. Every winding session on the couch, every walk in the park, every cuddle in the small hours is a moment you'll never get back.

Having your first baby is like nothing else and I envy what you've got to come.

Enjoy.

GLOSSARY

Pregnancy introduces you to an awful lot of new words, phrases and terms.

Most of the time you'll just nod and attempt to look wise and sympathetic as they are thrown at you, occasionally though you will need to understand what they mean.

Here are a few you might need.

A

Afterbirth

The placenta is commonly called the afterbirth once it has been delivered. Calling it afterbirth before that point can cause great offence, not only to the placenta in question, but placentas everywhere.

Amniocentesis

A diagnostic test used to determine possible genetic abnormalities. Amniotic fluid is withdrawn from the amniotic sac by inserting a hollow needle through the abdominal wall. The test itself carries a very small risk of miscarriage.

Amniotic fluid

A clear straw-coloured liquid in the amniotic sac in which the foetus grows. It cushions the baby against pressure and knocks, allows the baby to move around and grow without restriction, keeps the baby at a constant temperature, provides a barrier against infection and if the fact that your baby downs pint after pint of the stuff during its time in the womb is anything to go by, it tastes like cold German lager on a hot summer's day too.

Amniotic sac

Receptacle for the amber nectar called amniotic fluid.

Anal Armageddon

The dreaded double whammy of constipation and piles which all too often strikes down the pregnant lady.

Antenatal care

Medical care for a pregnant woman and her developing baby for the duration of the pregnancy – not care after the pregnancy, despite the fact that 'ante' sounds like it should mean after and not before. Why can't things just be simple?

Antenatal classes

A concept devised by 1970s sitcom writers as a means of generating awkward social situations for material. The initial purpose has long been forgotten and these classes are now used by many as a genuine way of learning about the birth.

Anterior position

The normal position for the baby to take up for late pregnancy and birth.

Apgar test

Test used straight after birth to assess a newborn baby's health by measuring five basic indicators of health: activity level, pulse, response to stimulation, appearance and respiration. The baby is given a score of 0, 1 or 2 on each indicator and the scores are added up to give an overall 'Apgar score' out of a possible 10.Essentially your child's first ever exam.

B

Babymoon

The holiday taken by many pregnant couples in the second trimester.

Baby blues

As is sometimes believed, the 'baby blues' is not a patronising term used by male doctors to describe full blown postnatal depression (p 261) – it refers specifically to a mild low point that many women experience three or four days after giving birth. Weepiness, mood swings, anxiety and/or unhappiness can all come about as a result of the dramatic drop in hormones after birth and from a feeling of anticlimax after actually giving birth.

Baby bomb

A nappy wearing incendiary device, which lands in the middle of your relationship and can cause substantial but not necessarily permanent damage.

Birth canal

The passage from the cervix through which the baby travels as he nears birth. The vagina to you and me.

Birthing centre

A hospital alternative for low-risk births where women can go through labour and delivery. Many contain the highest concentration of brightly coloured wipe-clean plastic furniture items anywhere on the planet.

Birth plan

A document that outlines how your partner would like to see the delivery progress, especially in terms of the treatment and pain relief she receives. The pregnancy equivalent of a letter to Santa.

Bishop's score

Method used to predict the success of inducing labour. Under no circumstances is this to be confused with the real ale of a similar name.

Blastocyst

The fertilised egg at around the stage when it enters the uterus. Also only a matter of time before it becomes the name of an ultra powerful multi-surface cleaner and grease remover.

Bloody show

A 'show' or 'bloody show' is the discharge of mucus tinged with blood that signifies the mucus plug dislodging as labour nears. Also what parents of a bygone age used to accuse their misbehaving offspring of making of them in public.

Braxton Hicks contractions

Joke contractions that maybe give the womb useful practice ahead of the main event, or exist purely as one of Mother Nature's jolly japes.

Breast pump

Portable milking parlour that allows breastfeeding mothers to extract milk from the breasts to either be given to the baby in a bottle or as a precautionary measure to avoid breast explosion as stocks increase to dangerous levels.

Breech position

When a baby is bottom down rather than head down in the uterus just before birth. Either the baby's bottom or feet would be born first causing painful havoc for its Mum.

C

C-section/caesarean section

A caesarean or c-section is when the baby is delivered through an incision in the mother's abdomen and then womb. It's used when a woman cannot give birth vaginally, if the baby is in distress or danger, or if the mother-to-be isn't overly keen on the agonies of natural childbirth and throws some money at it.

Carpal tunnel syndrome

Nothing to do with fishing and everything to do with the nerves in the wrist becoming compressed during pregnancy, resulting in a tingling, burning or numbness in the hands. If it persists after birth it directly affects a mother's ability to carry things at the exact time that she has the most important cargo of her entire life to cart about.

Cephalopelvic disproportion

As bad as it sounds. When a baby's head is too large to pass through the mother's pelvic opening because the baby is too large or in a bad position or if the mother's pelvis is small or abnormally shaped. Unsurprisingly, often results in delivery by caesarean section.

Cervical incompetence

Charming phrase to describe the condition where the cervix opens before a pregnancy has reached full term.

Cervical mucus method

The cervical mucus, or rhythm, method is a form of natural birth control which focuses on the consistency of the woman's cervical mucus. Thick and cloudy mucus indicates a time when conception is less likely, mucus similar to raw egg white signifies a time close to ovulation. Mucus that actually is raw egg white means someone up there is making a lemon meringue pie.

Cervix

A vital piece of pregnancy kit. The lower end or neck of the womb that leads into the vagina, and gradually opens during labour.

Chorionic villus sampling

Test for Down's syndrome carried out in early pregnancy. Cells lining the placenta are removed through the cervix or abdomen using a needle or catheter and tested.

Colostrum

The first liquid the breasts produce, ahead of breast milk itself. Rich in fats, protein, and antibodies, it protects the baby against infection and kick-starts the immune system. The original health drink.

Conception

The moment when sperm and egg meet, fall in love and join to form a single cell, before developing into an embryo and then a foetus.

Congenital problem

Any problem with a baby that is present from birth or has developed during pregnancy and is not inherited.

Contraction

The strong, rhythmic tightening of the muscles of the uterus as it opens up the cervix and pushes the baby out.

Crowning

When the baby's head can be seen at the opening of the vagina during labour. This occurrence is normally swiftly followed by the perilous question to the father – do you want to see, to which there is no correct answer.

D

D&C (dilation and curettage)

Surgical procedure in which the cervix is dilated and the lining of the uterus is scraped. Not nice.

Delivery room

A room in a hospital or birth centre that is equipped for childbirth, but tragically rarely sound-proofed.

Dilation

The gradual opening of the cervix during labour. At around 10cm the cervix is 'fully dilated' and you win a prize.

Doula

An individual specially trained to help during labour and after the birth of a baby or someone saying the name Nuala with a bad head cold.

Down's syndrome

The most common of many chromosomal abnormalities. Down's causes mild to severe learning disabilities, as well as other physical problems, such as heart defects.

Due date

The due date or estimated date of delivery is the date when a baby's birth is expected in the very loosest sense of the world. It is set by a doctor or midwife and is usually based on the first day of a woman's last period or their favourite number added to the date of their birthday.

Dystocia

A troublesome childbirth. Uterine dystocia occurs when contractions are not strong enough to deliver the baby. Shoulder dystocia happens when a baby's shoulders get stuck after the head has already been delivered.

E

Eclampsia

Eclampsia is a rare but deadly serious condition that affects women in late pregnancy. If pre-eclampsia (see p 261) is not treated, it can develop into eclampsia, which can cause convulsions and coma and may require emergency delivery of the baby.

Ectopic pregnancy

An early pregnancy worry causer. An ectopic occurs when a fertilised egg implants outside the uterus, usually in a fallopian tube. As there's not enough room for a baby to grow an ectopic must be surgically removed to prevent long-term damage.

ECV (external cephalic version)

The Heimlich manoeuvre for the unborn. Procedure done late in pregnancy, where a doctor manually attempts to move a baby in the breech position into the normal head-down position.

Effacement

This is the thinning and shortening of the cervix during early labour, often fruitfully called 'ripening'. During effacement, the cervix goes from more than 2.5cm thick to the width of a fag paper.

EFM (electronic foetal monitor)

A device used to monitor the progress and vital signs of a baby during labour. It records the baby's heartbeat and the woman's contractions.

Embryo

The medical term for a developing baby during the first eight weeks of pregnancy; after that, it is called a foetus, after that it's called Clive, or Janice or whatever unfortunate moniker you give the poor mite.

Engagement

Engagement is when the foetus descends into the pelvic cavity before delivery. Also known as lock and load.

Engorgement

This term describes the breasts becoming full, swollen and tender, usually sometime between two days and a week after birth, when a mother's milk comes in. As if they didn't have enough on their plate.

Epidural

A form of pain relief for labour in which anaesthetic is injected around the spinal cord. That's got to hurt. The lower body is numbed and pain is decreased or eliminated altogether.

Episiotomy

A surgical cut in the never, never land between the vagina and the anus made to enlarge the vaginal opening and get the baby out of there without tearing the ladies' bits to smithereens.

F

Face presentation

Baby comes into the birth canal face first, but this is rare. Most babies born like this pursue a career in acting.

Fallopian tube

The two tubes, one each side of the womb that act as a water slide for each month's egg(s).

Foetal alcohol syndrome

The physical and mental birth defects caused by a baby's mother consuming large amounts of alcohol during pregnancy.

Foetal distress

During labour slow heartbeat or absence of foetal movement are carefully watched for throughout. If a foetus's life is believed to be in danger the baby is usually delivered as soon as possible.

Foetal monitor

The device used to track a foetus's heartbeat and a woman's uterine contractions during labour. Looks a bit like Wonderwoman's belt.

Foetal presentation

Not a 15-minute PowerPoint on what gives amniotic fluid its beautiful flavour, but the position of the baby – such as feet down (breech) or head down (vertex) – inside the womb.

Foetal-maternal exchange

The transfer of life-giving nutrients from the mother to the baby and the transfer of waste from the baby to his mother. This very one-sided transaction continues for many years.

Foetus

The term for a baby after eight weeks of development. Before that the developing baby is called an embryo.

Folic acid

The queen of all the pregnancy supplements. Folic acid has been shown to reduce the incidence of neural tube defects such as spina bifida and a horrific sounding condition called anencephaly, a partially or completely missing brain.

Fontanelle

Soft spots on a baby's head which essentially allow his skull to move and flex during birth so he stands a cat in hell's chance of squeezing out of there. Fontanelles are usually hardened by the time your child is two years.

Forceps delivery

When a giant pair of medieval looking tongs are used to 'ease' the baby's head through the birth canal during delivery. Never has an instrument looked less suited to be used on the soft flesh of a baby's tiny head.

Fraternal twins

Born at the same time from two different eggs they are no more genetically similar than siblings born during different pregnancies. Nothing annoys fraternal twins more than repeatedly describing them as identical. Try it.

Full-term

A baby is considered full-term if born between 38 and 42 weeks' gestation.

Fundus

The upper, rounded portion of the womb. Also, maker of crispy pancakes.

G

Genitals

Surely you know this? The external sex organs: the penis and testicles in a male and the labia in a female.

Gestation

The period in which a baby is carried in the womb; full-term gestation is between 38 and 42 weeks.

Grasping reflex

A newborn baby's innate reflex which sees it grab at an object, such as a finger, when it touches their hand. The reflex lasts until a baby is three to four months old, and has been linked to our evolutionary past which saw our ancestral young gripping tightly to their mother's fur as they moved through the tree canopy.

H

Haemorrhoids

There's no easy way of saying this, but pregnant women are much more susceptible to piles. I know, I know, as if they didn't have enough to worry about.

Health visitor

A registered nurse with qualifications in obstetrics and midwifery, who visits mothers and babies at home after the birth. The 'niceness' or otherwise of one's health visitor becomes a conversation staple among new parents in the first few weeks of parenthood.

Hormone

A messenger from one cell (or group of cells) to another. Hormones use chemicals to stimulate or slow down various functions throughout the body. They are also to blame for the vast majority of pregnancy symptoms that women experience during pregnancy and become the generic scapegoat for much of what occurs across the nine months. The levels of some hormones in a pregnant woman are increased by more than 10 times the normal levels, and recent research also suggests that the male partner's hormones fluctuate at the same time too.

Hormonal henchmen

The collective term for the chemical bandits who terrorise pregnant women, bringing on such delights as indigestion, constipation, haemorrhoids and morning sickness. Progesterone, oestrogen, oxytocin, relaxin and a squad of endorphins act as the leaders of the gang.

Hysterectomy

Surgical removal of the womb – often threatened by mother in the immediate aftermath of labour.

I

Identical twins

Offspring born at the same time who look exactly alike – a single fertilised egg splits early in development and becomes two separate foetuses.

Implantation

Occurs when a fertilised egg attaches itself to the lining of the womb and the whole crazy business kicks off.

In vitro fertilisation

An assisted conception treatment in which eggs and sperm are mixed in a laboratory. Up to three developing embryos can then be transferred to the woman's uterus with the aim of achieving pregnancy. Not cheap.

Incubator

A box-like piece of kit in which premature babies are kept at a constant temperature.

Induced labour

Labour started using a medication rather than being naturally begun.

Infant

Technically, a child between one month and one year of age.

Infant mortality

Refers to death of babies during the first year of their life.

Intrauterine growth restriction

The slow growth of a foetus in the uterus, possibly resulting in a low birth weight baby.

J

Jaundice

Too much bilirubin in the blood. Jaundice manifests as a yellow tinge to a baby's skin. Newborn jaundice usually begins on the second or third day of life and starts disappearing when the baby is 7–10 days old. It can be sometimes corrected by a special UV light treatment.

K

Kick count

Record of how often a pregnant woman feels her baby move; used to evaluate foetal well-being.

L

Labour

The process of childbirth, from the moment the cervix begins to dilate, to the delivery of the baby and the placenta.

Labour suite/room

The labour suite is where a woman goes through labour and delivers her baby. Never has the word suite been so misplaced.

Lactation

The production of breast milk.

Lanugo

Downy-like, fine hair on a foetus and newborn baby.

Latching on

A phrase you will use one hundred thousand times in the first week of being a parent. To 'latch on' is the notionally in-built, but seemingly bloody difficult, art of the baby suckling from the breast without causing his mother to endure agony after agony.

Leg cramps

Having a woman in the eighth month of pregnancy wake up beside you in the middle of the night and scream out in real pain is not good for the nerves. No one knows why cramps occur more during pregnancy, but they do. Maybe it's just someone having a laugh at our expense?

Let-down

Let-down is the release of milk in a breastfeeding mother as the baby starts to suckle. Can also be what you become in the early weeks of fatherhood, despite you doing your very best to be helpful and supportive.

Lightening

The feeling a woman gets when the foetus positions itself lower in the pelvic cavity during the last throws of pregnancy. For thunder, please see wind, p 97.

Linea nigra

The dark line that often develops during pregnancy, running from below the breasts and over the abdomen and navel.

Lochia

Vaginal discharge of mucus, blood and tissue, which can continue for up to six weeks after delivery. You and your partner may well coin your own term for this delightful phenomenon.

Low birth weight

A full-term baby who weighs less than 5.5lbs at birth.

M

Mask of pregnancy

Increased pigmentation under each eye during pregnancy.

Manager Mum

Often the result of a career woman adjusting to the full-time job of bringing up baby. Routine, rules and reprimands can result.

Maternal mortality

The death of a mother at any point during pregnancy, birth or the year following delivery. Tragically, the biggest cause of maternal death in the UK is suicide.

Maternity leave

Paid or unpaid time off work after a mother has given birth or adopted a child.

Meconium

The dark, tar-like substance that forms a newborn's first bowel movement. The next one looks like chicken korma.

Metabolic rate

The amount of oxygen consumed by a pregnant woman when she is at rest is her basal metabolism. The rate begins to rise during the third month of pregnancy and can double by the time of delivery. She is one busy lady.

Midwife

Midwives provide care to women during pregnancy, labour, birth, and for the first few days after too. A friendly, caring and sympathetic midwife is a thing of beauty and a joy forever. A horrible one is a curse.

Milia

Tiny, harmless white spots on a newborn that usually disappear by themselves, after you've worried about them for 48 hours solid. This is a pretty fair reflection of how your life is going to be for at least the next year.

Miscarriage

The involuntary expulsion of a foetus before the 24th week. After that point the loss of a pregnancy is called a stillbirth.

Morning sickness

Not necessarily in the morning and not necessarily sickness, but a combination of food and smell aversions, nausea and occasional vomiting, in the early weeks of pregnancy.

Mucus plug

As its name suggests a plug made from mucus which seals the entrance to the cervix during pregnancy.

Mumnesia

The forgetfulness phenomenon that afflicts pregnant women. See Hormonal henchmen for main culprits.

N

Natural childbirth

Labour and delivery short on medical intervention, high on pain.

NCT

The National Childbirth Trust – providers of antenatal classes and pre- and post-pregnancy support. A Godsend for some, a herbal tea hell for others.

Neonatal

The first six weeks after birth.

Neonatal intensive care unit

Specialist unit for the care of seriously ill or premature babies.

Nuchal translucency screening

Nerve-wracking ultrasound procedure in which the doctor measures the space behind the baby's neck. Combined with blood test results this measures the probability of a baby having Down's syndrome.

O

Obstetrician

Specialist in pregnancy, childbirth and the immediate aftermath.

Oestrogen

A hormone produced by the ovaries that regulates the reproductive cycle and plays a whole host of other roles throughout a pregnant woman's body.

Oligospermia

Scrabble players word for low sperm count.

Ovaries

The female sex glands – also called gonads – situated on either side of the womb and which produce the key female hormones and the all-important eggs.

Ovulation

When a mature egg is released from the ovaries into the fallopian tubes – the time around when a woman is most likely to conceive and most likely to think that you look quite nice in that shirt.

Oxytocin

A hormone that controls contractions and stimulates the flow of breast milk. A synthetic version is often used to induce labour.

P

Perineum

The small, landing-strip-type area between the vagina and anus which is where an episiotomy, if required, is performed.

Perineal massage

Complex rubbing motion, similar to the hold used on a bowling ball, performed using oils on the perineum to try to prevent tearing during childbirth.

Pethidine

Pain-relieving drug used during childbirth. A member of the morphine family, it can turn labour into a psychedelic scene from *Apocalypse Now*. It's usually given as an injection into the thigh and can cause drowsiness and nausea; there is some evidence that it can affect the baby too.

Placenta

A bagpipe-like organ that grows in the womb during pregnancy to provide nutrients for the foetus.

Placenta praevia

Not a new Toyota people carrier, but a condition where the placenta attaches itself to the lower part of the uterus and develops in a low-lying position.

Polycystic ovary syndrome

A condition that prevents a woman's eggs from receiving the right growth signal from her brain, meaning her eggs don't mature and are not released. As the eggs die, their follicles turn into cysts which can then cause the ovaries to enlarge, sometimes to the size of a grapefruit.

Posterior position

Birth position where the baby's spine is against the mother's back – sometimes called back to back or simply the awkward little bugger position.

Postnatal depression

A serious condition, not to be confused with the baby blues (p 243) that many women suffer from in the first few days after pregnancy. Characterised by sadness, impatience and an inability to care for or connect with the baby. Medical help should be sought ASAP if this is suspected.

Pre-eclampsia

Often occurring late in pregnancy, pre-eclampsia results in high blood pressure and protein in the urine and can lead to eclampsia (p 248), where the mother goes into convulsions. Pre-eclampsia is thought to be due to a problem with the placenta.

Pregnancy-induced hypertension

A common condition in which a woman's blood pressure is temporarily elevated. It usually happens during the last trimester. No one has done any research as to whether the father-to-be's blood pressure rises during the final trimester too – but I'd say so.

Pregnancy pina colada

The heady and potent mix of hormones that combine to make pregnancy such a joy for femalekind.

Premature baby

A baby born before 37 weeks of gestation.

Primary maternal preoccupation

The psychoanalytical term for the unbreakable bond between mother and child that cements in place during the first few weeks of parenthood.

Primitive reflexes

A newborn baby's involuntary reflexes that often disappear after the first few weeks. Many, for example the automatic closing of the hand when the palm is touched (p 252), have been linked back to different stages of our evolutionary journey as a species.

Progesterone

Female hormone produced in the ovaries that works with oestrogen to regulate the reproductive cycle.

Prolactin

Hormone that activates a mother's milk-producing glands. The delivery of the placenta is the signal to start producing prolactin.

Prolonged labour

The official term for a long, difficult labour that is still going after 18–24 hours. The unofficial term, which you may hear used by your partner is – absolute fucking torture.

Q

Quickening

Quaint term for the first movement of the baby felt by the mother-to-be. The quaintness dissipates somewhat as movements become more forceful later on.

R

Respiratory distress syndrome

A relatively common but scary as hell condition in premature babies in which the air sacs in the lungs collapse because they don't contain enough of an essential substance called surfactant. Most babies recover when given increased oxygen.

Rhesus incompatibility

When a baby inherits a blood type from his father which is different from and incompatible with his mother's. Blood tests will usually determine if there is a problem ahead of delivery.

Rooting reflex

A baby's automatic reaction to turn his head and start sucking when his cheek is stroked. Lingers for many decades in some men's cases.

S

Show

A 'show' or 'bloody show' if you are feeling annoyed, is the mucusy, blood tinged discharge that occurs when the mucus plug comes away as labour nears.

Sonographer

Medical professionals who operate the ultrasound scanning machine. A skilled sonographer will be able to give you a real insight into your baby's womb world. An unskilled one will be able to show you a satellite map of the low pressure front over the Orkneys.

Squat bar

A U-shaped bar attached to a birthing bed to allow a labouring woman to squat when she's ready to push the baby out. Not the place to hang your coat up when you arrive.

Stillbirth

The loss of a pregnancy after 24 weeks.

Stretch marks

Marks in the skin caused by rapidly growing tissue – a common side effect of pregnancy. The answer to the question 'Are those stretch marks?', as asked by a pregnant woman, is always no.

Symbiotic stage

The early and very close relationship between a mother and her newborn. Not to be confused with the probiotic stage which is a father's massive early pregnancy heartburn brought on by too much wine and not enough sleep.

T

Toxoplasmosis

A parasitic and nasty infection carried by cats' faeces and uncooked meat that can cause stillbirth or miscarriage if a woman contracts it for the first time during pregnancy. Avoiding litter trays and washing hands thoroughly after handling meat are a must when expecting.

Transition

Phase of labour in which the cervix fully dilates like the opening of an enormous telescope observatory's roof.

Trimester

A trimester is a period of three months. Pregnancy consists of three trimesters. That's nine months. Is that clear?

U

Ultrasound

High-frequency sound waves used to create a moving image of your baby in the womb.

Umbilical cord

The structure that connects a foetus to its life-giving, if ugly, mate the placenta. The cord, which looks and feels like those bloated French sausages that you always avoid in the hypermarket while on holiday there, is cut after the delivery. Later on, the stump end left attached to your baby, which has been slowly dying and giving off the unmistakable stench of rotting flesh, eventually falls off revealing your baby's belly button.

Uterus

See womb.

V

Vaginal birth

When a baby is delivered via the birth canal rather than the sun roof.

Varicose veins

Just like its close cousin piles, varicose veins strike pregnant women thanks to the hormone progesterone causing blood vessels in the vein walls to relax.

Ventouse extraction

Procedure in which a suction cup is placed on the baby's head to assist the baby's passage through the birth canal. If that sounds like a nice way of saying that the baby is yanked out of your partner's vagina using a plunger, it's because it pretty much is.

Vernix caseosa

A greasy substance which covers the baby in the womb. It is used like goose fat by channel swimmers to form a barrier as they float around in fluid for nine months.

Very low birth weight

A very low birth weight baby is one weighing under 3.3lb (1.5kg) at birth.

W

Witch's milk

The milk sometimes produced by a newborn's breasts at birth. Don't run out of the delivery room screaming though, it's a hormonal condition that disappears after a few days.

Womb

See uterus.

X

X-ray

Not really relevant, but makes more sense than seeing xylophone here.

Y

Yellow body

The yellow mass of cells that forms in the follicle of the ovary after the release of an egg. The yellow body acts on the lining of the uterus, which becomes spongy, ready to receive a fertilised egg.

Z

Zygote

Medical term for a newly fertilised egg on its way down to implant into the uterus.

References

1. BBC News. River 'pollution' sparks fertility fears. 17 March 2002.
Available at: http://news.bbc.co.uk/1/hi/uk/1877162.stm

2. 'Worried hubbies secretly fear Junior not theirs' *Gainesville Sun*. 4
January 1987.

3. Mothers 35 plus. Losing a baby. 1998–2009. Available at: www.
mothers35plus.co.uk/losing.htm

4. BBC News. Painkillers 'may boost miscarriage risk'. 15 August 2003.
Available at: http://news.bbc.co.uk/1/hi/health/3148861.stm

5. The Ectopic Pregnancy Trust. Available at: www.ectopic.org.uk/
medical_information/faq.htm

6. The Baby Website.com. Pregnancy ruins your love life. November
2008. Available at: www.thebabywebsite.com/article.1677.Pregnancy_
Ruins_Your_Love_Life.htm

7. Netmums. Lets talk about sex (after kids): Survey Results. 2010.
Available at: www.netmums.com/homelife/Lets_Talk_about_sex_
after_kids__Survey_Results.1937/

8. Suite 101.com. Expectant fathers. Available at: www.suite101.com/
lesson.cfm/19164/2815/2

9. California Birth Defects Monitoring Program. Work, hobbies
and gastroschisis. April 1999. Available at: www.cbdmp.org/pdf/
gastroworkhobbies.pdf

10. BBC News. Men suffer from phantom pregnancy. 14 June 2007.
Available at: http://news.bbc.co.uk/1/hi/health/6751709.stm

11. Evolution and human behaviour. 2009. Available at:
www.ehbonline.org/article/S1090-5138(99)00042-2/abstract

12. BBC News. Pregnancy cravings 'on the rise'. 28 April 2008.

Available at: http://news.bbc.co.uk/1/hi/health/7370524.stm

13. New Scientist. Pregnant women get that shrinking feeling. 11 January 1997. Available at: www.newscientist.com/article/mg15320640.400-pregnant-women-get-that-shrinking-feeling.html

14. *Telegraph*. Mumnesia is a medical fact, say scientists. 6 March 2008. Available at: www.telegraph.co.uk/earth/earthnews/3335107/Mumnesia-is-a-medical-fact-say-scientists.html

15. British Journal of Psychiatry: Cognition in pregnancy and motherhood. Available at: http://bjp.rcpsych.org/cgi/content/abstract/196/2/126

16. BBC Features. Womb music. Available at: www.bbc.co.uk/print/music/parents/features/wombmusic.shtml

17. Behind the Name. Names and behaviour. 1996–2009. Available at: www.behindthename.com/articles/1.php

18. Behind the Name. Names and personality. 1996–2009. Available at: www.behindthename.com/articles/2.php

19. Times Online. Jack and Olivia most popular baby names. 9 September 2009. Available at: www.timesonline.co.uk/tol/news/uk/article6825857.ece

20. Fatherhood Institute. Men who respond to impending fatherhood by examining their own childhood produce happier children. December 2003. Available at: www.fatherhoodinstitute.org/index.php?id=2&cID=263

21. Fathers To Be. What good are dads - key findings. Available at: www.fatherstobe.org/What%20good%20are%20dads.pdf

22. BBC News. Fathers urged to bath baby. 7 November 2001. Available at: http://news.bbc.co.uk/1/hi/health/1642676.stm

23. *Sunday Morning Herald*. Ante-natal classes in pubs for men. 12 October 2009. Available at: http://news.smh.com.au/breaking-news-national/antenatal-classes-in-pubs-for-men-20091012-gskh.html

24. *Guardian*. Natural childbirth techniques no better than standard antenatal classes. 27 May 2009. Available at: www.guardian.co.uk/lifeandstyle/besttreatments/2009/may/27/natural-childbirth-techniques-no-better-than-standard-antenatal-classes

25. Desmond M. *Babywatching*. London: Jonathan Cape, 1991.

26. Hill A. You thought children would make you happy? Not really – just poorer. *The Observer*. 16 November 2003. Available at: http://www.guardian.co.uk/society/2003/nov/16/childrensservices.childreninbritain

27. Evenson RJ, Simon RW. Clarifying the relationship between parenthood and depression. *Journal of Health and Social Behaviour* December 2005; 46:341–58.

28. Study by Cowan PA, Professor of Psychology, Cowan CP, Research Psychologist, University of California at Berkeley, 1985 and Belsky J, Professor of Human Development at Pennsylvania State University, 1988.

29. Winnicott D. *Primary maternal preoccupation, through paediatrics to psychoanalysis*. London: Hogarth, 1956.

30. *The Washington Independent*. DOJ advice on sleep deprivation varied widely. 9 March 2009. Available at: http://washingtonindependent.com/57617/doj-advice-on-sleep-deprivation-varied-widely

31. Preemie Survival Foundation. You can help premature babies and families. Available at: www.preemiesurvival.org/

32. BBC News. More premature babies surviving. 3 June 2009. Available at: http://news.bbc.co.uk/1/hi/health/8078911.stm

33. Nuffield Council on Bioethics. Critical care decisions in fetal and neonatal medicine: ethical issues. 16 November 2006. Available at: www.nuffieldbioethics.org/go/ourwork/neonatal/publication_406. html

34. EPICure. 2008. Available at: www.epicure.ac.uk/

35. BBC News. Working increases risk to pregnancy. 17 April 2002. Available at: http://news.bbc.co.uk/1/hi/health/1932578.stm

36. Simpson M, Parsons M, Greenwood J, *et al.* Raspberry leaf in pregnancy: its safety and efficacy in labour. *Journal of Midwifery and Women's Health* 2001;46(2):51–9.

37. *Guardian.* Men should 'stay away from childbirth'. 18 October 2009. Available at: www.guardian.co.uk/lifeandstyle/2009/oct/18/men-birth-labour-baby

38. Fatherhood Institute. Fathers at the birth and after: impact on mothers. 29 September 2007. Available at: www.fatherhoodinstitute. org/index.php?id=2&cID=578

39. *Guardian.* It's good for women to suffer the pain of a natural birth, says medical chief. 12 July 2009. Available at: www.guardian.co.uk/lifeandstyle/2009/jul/12/pregnancy-pain-natural-birth-yoga

40. *Guardian.* It's good for women to suffer the pain of a natural birth, says medical chief. 12 July 2009. Available at: www.guardian.co.uk/lifeandstyle/2009/jul/12/pregnancy-pain-natural-birth-yoga

41. *Herald Scotland.* Swearing may be a blessing, not a curse. 18 July 2009. Available at: www.heraldscotland.com/swearing-may-be-a-blessing-not-a-curse-1.829935

42. NCT. Concern over maternity statistics. 30 April 2009. Available at: www.nctpregnancyandbabycare.com/press-office/press-releases/view/144

Index

SAVE MONEY
RAISING YOUR CHILD

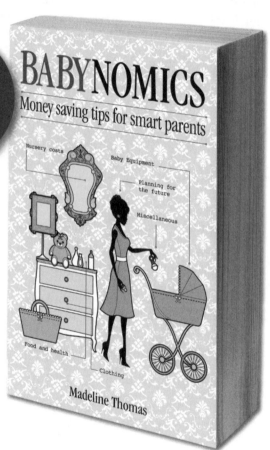

Special Offer
15% off
Only
£8.49

BABYNOMICS
Money saving tips for smart parents

Nursery costs
Baby Equipment
Planning for the future
Miscellaneous
Food and health
Clothing

Madeline Thomas

- ❧ What NOT to waste your money on
- ❧ Shopping tips from bargain hunting parents
- ❧ Building a nest egg for your family